VAGUS NERVE

Activate your vagus nerve Activate your life!

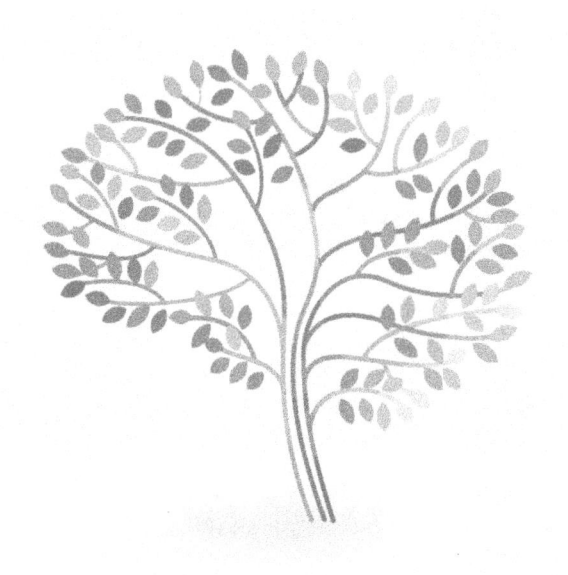

Robert Dickens

Table of Contents

TABLE OF CONTENTS 2

INTRODUCTION 4

THE AUTONOMIC NERVOUS SYSTEM 7

- THE EVOLUTION OF THE NERVOUS SYSTEM 9
- THE STRUCTURE OF THE NERVOUS SYSTEM 14
- THE CENTRAL NERVOUS SYSTEM 15
- THE PERIPHERAL NERVOUS SYSTEM. 16
- THE AUTONOMIC NERVOUS SYSTEM 17
- FUNCTIONS OF THE NERVOUS SYSTEM 23
- THE CRANIAL NERVES 27

THE VAGUS NERVE 31

- THE STRUCTURE OF THE VAGUS NERVE 31
- THE FUNCTIONS OF THE VAGUS NERVE 34
- THE ROLE OF THE VAGUS NERVE IN GOOD HEALTH 40

THE POLYVAGAL THEORY 45

DISORDERS ASSOCIATED WITH VAGUS NERVE MALFUNCTION 52

- SYMPTOMS OF VAGUS NERVE DYSFUNCTION 53
- INFLAMMATION 59
- THE ROLE OF THE VAGUS NERVE IN INFLAMMATION 63
- PHYSICAL DISORDERS 64
- MENTAL DISORDERS 75

VAGUS NERVE STIMULATION — 84

- VAGAL TONE — 87
- ACTIVATING THE VAGUS NERVE — 92
- ACCESSING THE HEALING POWER OF THE VAGUS NERVE — 96

MEDITATION — 112

- INCREASING PARASYMPATHETIC RESPONSES THROUGH MEDITATION — 114
- MEDITATION TECHNIQUES — 116
- THE WIM HOF METHOD — 128

EXERCISES TO ENHANCE VAGUS FUNCTION — 135

- SPECIFIC YOGA POSES — 136
- BREATHING EXERCISES — 143
- USEFUL TIPS — 147

CONCLUSION — 154

Introduction

The following chapters will discuss the amazing self-healing powers of the body and how to activate it. A balanced or homeostatic state in the body is required to facilitate optimal organ function, and ultimately, good health. This homeostatic state is facilitated by two opposing systems of the autonomic nervous system that have opposing responses, and therefore, balance each other out. These are the sympathetic nervous system and the parasympathetic nervous system.

When either the sympathetic or parasympathetic nervous system is overstimulated for extended periods of time, organ function is disrupted, leading to physical and psychological disorders in the body. This is where the Vagus nerve comes in. The Vagus nerve, being the largest cranial nerve, is widespread throughout the body and has both motor and sensory control on various body organs. This crucial nerve ensures that balance is maintained in the body by inhibiting prolonged fight or flight responses from the sympathetic system.

While the vagus nerve functions naturally, age and other stress factors can inhibit its activity leading to a decreased vagal tone. This, therefore, means that we need to equip ourselves with the knowledge on how to stimulate and activate the vagus nerve in order to reap its self-healing benefits. Not only is the vagus nerve effective in the prevention of certain conditions, but it is also an effective therapy in the management of chronic inflammation and the resulting disorders such as rheumatoid arthritis.

By learning how to hack into the powers of the vagus nerve, you will significantly improve your health and facilitate a natural pathway that the body can use to naturally heal and repair itself. Good health stems from in-depth knowledge of how our body works and what we can do to ensure that important elements such as the Vagus nerve are consistently stimulated and active.

There are plenty of books on this subject on the market, thanks for choosing this one! Every effort was made to ensure it is full of as much useful information as possible. Please enjoy it!

Chapter 1

The Autonomic Nervous System

Cindy is out for a walk in the park. It's a pleasant summer morning, and the heat has lulled her into a comfortable semi-daze. She is lost in thought and does not notice the rattling in the bushes around the corner. As she draws up to the bush, a huge dog rears its head out of the bush and lets out a loud bark. Startled, she leaps back eyes wide and terrified and lets out a shriek. The dog runs off, and she is left bent over, clutching her thudding chest as she tries to catch her breath.

At one point or another, we have all been startled or scared. Think of watching a scary movie, coming upon a particularly large bug, or your friend jumping out from a dark corner and yelling "boo!" Our reactions are almost always the same when we are frightened or startled; our heart starts beating rapidly, our breathing quickens, and our eyes open wider. But have you ever stopped to consider how these reflexes come about? You never actively think, "Oh, am I going to scream now?" or "Am I going to increase my heart rate?" These things all happen instinctively without conscious control or thought, and you find yourself reacting even before you know what is happening.

Our bodies have natural self-defense mechanisms that function by identifying changes in our environment and eliciting an appropriate response to these potential dangers in our surroundings. When a baby touches a hot stove, they will immediately withdraw their hand. They do not need to know what fire is or understand the concept of heat; they will simply react to the potential harm in their environment by reflexive instinct.

This means that the body is equipped to defend itself without cognitive input. Without these natural reflexes, we would not be able to get ourselves out of harm's way, and therefore, these natural defense mechanisms are crucial for survival. These natural responses are facilitated by a system in our body that is responsible for the sensation of stimuli, response to the stimuli, and the regulation of our motor responses. This system is responsible for receiving information from the environment around us (sensation) and generating the appropriate reaction to that information (motor response). This system is referred to as the nervous system.

The Evolution of the Nervous System

The survival of any particular species is dependent on its ability to safeguard itself long enough to pass on its genes to the next generation. From the beginning of time, animals have developed and evolved complex survival mechanisms to ensure longevity and species propagation. One of these mechanisms is the flight or fight response that is regulated by the autonomic nervous system.

The fight or flight mechanism of the body evolved as a means to enable the body to not only detect danger but respond appropriately to it in order to avoid coming to any harm. This fight or flight response is part of the sympathetic responses of the autonomic nervous system. When you are in danger or facing an imminent attack, your body needs extra reserves of energy to enable you to either fight the threat or flee from it. To avail this extra energy to the body, the sympathetic nervous system initiates mechanisms that ensure your heart is pumping more blood, your cells have more oxygen, and your muscles are primed.

This autonomous nervous system has, over time, played a major role in the survival of generations of all animal species. These automated responses are the ones that will enable a deer to outrun a lion when it is being hunted and will cause your heart to beat faster and your breathing to become rapid when you are in danger. Without these fight or flight system, our lives would be woefully short because we would not be able to protect ourselves from harm.

One of the main elements that facilitate the fight and flight responses is the hormone adrenaline. This hormone is secreted in the adrenal glands, and once it is released, it has an effect on the heartbeat, respiration rate, vision, and sweat glands. You may have heard of someone experiencing an adrenaline rush; this refers to a state of intense stimulation of the body. Generally, adrenaline has the following effects on your body:

- Increasing the heart rate, which will cause you to feel your heart beating faster in your chest.

- Redirecting blood toward the muscles. This, in turn, increases the energy in the muscles, and you may even notice that your muscles start to shake or tremble.

- Relaxing the airways, which, in turn, has the effect of increasing the oxygen flow to the muscles.

- Widening of the eyes which is meant to allow more light into the pupils and enhance vision.

- It decreases the body's ability to feel pain. Ever noticed how, when you are running from something, you do not feel any pain in your muscles or chest until the danger is passed? This is one of the effects of adrenaline.

- Increasing strength or stamina. When adrenaline is realized in the body, it increases your strength, and this is why you find that when you are scared, you can lift things you ordinarily wouldn't or fight off people much bigger than you.

- Sharpens mental focus. You will find that your mental clarity is much sharper when you are in a dangerous situation, and you tend to think faster.

From the most prehistoric organisms which lacked the complex brain and nervous system development evident in animals today, they were as capable of this fight or flight response as the current species are. Many species of animals still use this instinct to survive. However, while humans still have this fight or flight response, it is much more evolved and has a wider application than simply escaping danger when it comes to humans.

Stress or danger, for most humans, takes on more complex definitions than simply the threat of bodily harm or loss of life. When an animal is trying to survive in the jungle, its survival instinct is centered around finding food and outrunning predators. When it comes to humans, our causes of danger or stress are more varied and wider. Stress for us comes in the form of our professions or work, relationships, and health issues.

We still use our fight or flight response, just in a different way. For instance, when you have a major presentation at work or have to speak in public for the first time, your increased anxiety will trigger the fight or flight response, and you will notice that your heart rate increases, you start to sweat, and your breathing becomes shallow. What this means is that your body does not know the difference between danger from a lion chasing you or your anxiety at giving a speech, in both these cases, the fight and flight mode is activated.

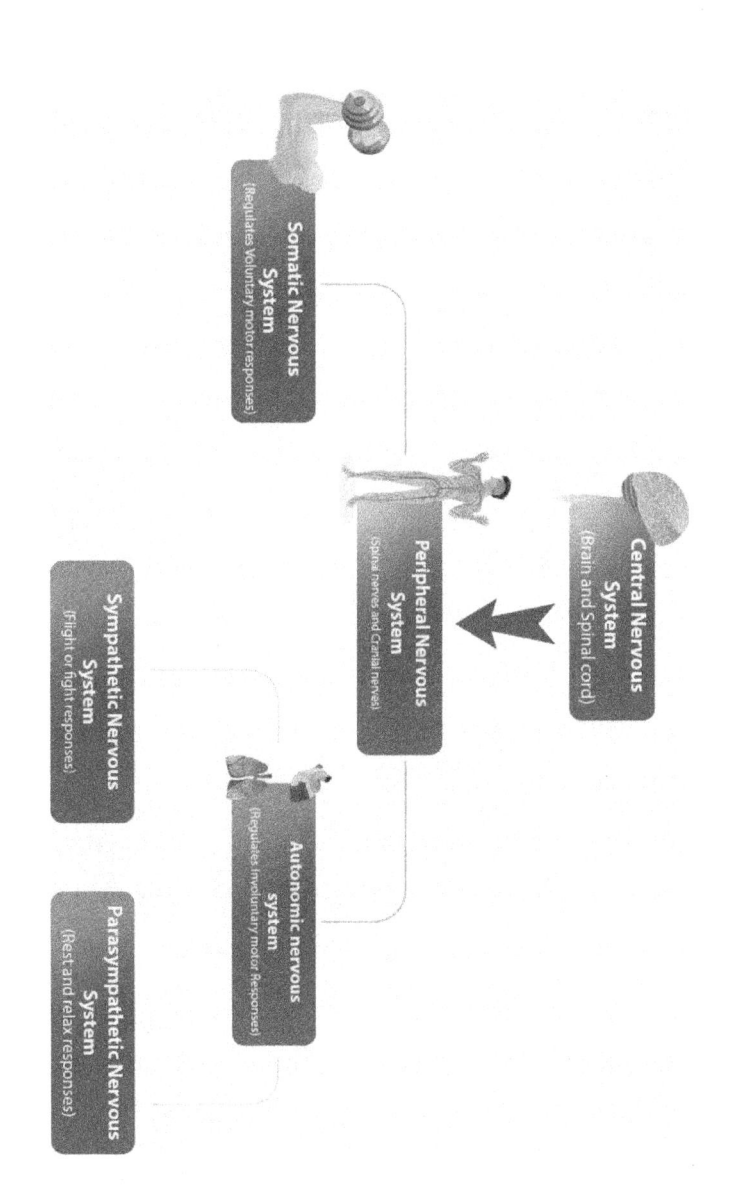

Nervous System Organization

- **Central Nervous System** (Brain and Spinal cord)
  - **Peripheral Nervous System** (Spinal nerves and Cranial nerves)
    - **Somatic Nervous System** (Regulates Voluntary motor responses)
    - **Autonomic nervous system** (Regulates Involuntary motor Responses)
      - **Sympathetic Nervous System** (Flight or fight responses)
      - **Parasympathetic Nervous System** (Rest and relax responses)

The Structure of the Nervous System

The structure of the nervous system is complex. The nervous system is made up of various branches, each with their unique roles and functions in the body.

The nervous system conveys signals between various parts of the body. This system is comprised of specialized cells that are referred to as neurons. Neurons are specialized nerve cells that act as signal conductors through which organs and cells in the body can communicate with each other by sending signals to each other. The neurons conduct signals in the form of electrochemical waves that are received as neurotransmitters. The neurotransmitters are released at synaptic junctions, and any cell that receives the synaptic signal is either activated or inhibited.

Neurons typically form interlinked chains and networks that are responsible for the way we perceive our environment and respond to it. These functions, of sensation and response, are coordinated in the brain and spinal cord, which form the central nervous system. This system is further divided into the peripheral nervous system and the autonomic nervous system.

The Central Nervous System

The brain and the spinal cord are the major structures that make up the central nervous system. The brain is surrounded by a protective layer referred to as the cranium and encased in the skull. The spinal cord is continuous with the brain and starts from the base of the skull extending through the vertebrae to terminate at the lumbar vertebrae.

The central nervous system is composed of both white and grey matter. In the white matter, it consists of nerve fibers referred to as axons. The axons form part of the structure of neurons. The axons in the white matter are insulated by myelin cells, which function as support cells for the axons. The myelin cells are lipid-rich, and hence, responsible for the white appearance that lends its name to the white matter.

In the gray matter, neurons and unmyelinated fibers are the main constituents. The lack of myelin in the gray matter leads to its darker appearance hence the name gray matter. Glial cells are present in both the white and gray matter.

Information is transmitted to the brain through the spinal tracts present in the spinal cord.

The Peripheral Nervous System.

The peripheral nervous system is one of the branches of the central nervous system and consists of cranial nerves and spinal nerves. The cranial nerves originate from the brain, while the spinal nerves originate from the spinal cord. The peripheral nervous system links the brain to the arms, legs, hands, and feet through sensory neurons, ganglia, and nerves.

Voluntary control of body movements is carried out by the somatic nervous system, which forms part of the peripheral nervous system. Conscious perception and voluntary motor responses are controlled by the somatic nervous system. Reflexes such as recoiling from a perceived threat are motor responses that are initiated by the somatic nervous system. Voluntary motor responses are usually a result of the contraction of skeletal muscle.

Signals from our major senses, such as sight, smell, or touch, are conveyed to the brain through the spinal cord by the sensory nervous system which forms part of the peripheral nervous system. When we come into contact with external stimuli through our senses, such as touch, this signal is transmitted to the brain through the spinal code. This means that the nervous system functions in the sensation of different stimuli that we routinely come into contact with and in the generation of an appropriate response to the stimuli.

The Autonomic nervous System

The involuntary physiological processes that occur in our bodies, such as breathing, blood flow, digestive processes, and the pumping of the heart are all regulated by the autonomic nervous system. This means that the autonomic nervous system regulates involuntary body responses.

These involuntary responses are characterized by the contraction of smooth muscles, activation of glands, and the regulation of cardiac muscles. The functions of the autonomic nervous system thus range from respiration and cardiac function to reflexes such as coughing and sneezing,

When you take a stroll outside on a hot afternoon, you will notice that you are sweating more than you would if it was cool or if you were indoors in an airconditioned room. Sweating is an example of one of the involuntary responses that are initiated by the autonomic nervous system. When the body starts feeling too hot, the autonomic nerves system triggers the sweat glands to produce more sweat as a self-cooling mechanism.

A jogger on his morning run will notice his heart rate speeding up and increasing with the intensity of the physical exercise. When you jog, your muscles need more oxygen to deal with the exertion of the physical exercise; this means that the autonomic nervous system has to innervate the heart muscles to pump faster and, as a result, supply more oxygen to the tissues.

All these processes are continuously occurring in our bodies as we go about our day so that we can adjust according to our surroundings in such a way that the body is maintained in the ideal homeostatic state that is necessary for organ function. For example, if you needed to run but your heart was not stimulated by the autonomic nervous system then, your muscles would not receive the added oxygen needed to facilitate the exercise, and you would be out of breath in no time.

It is, therefore, important to note that without the autonomic nervous system, our body functions would be impaired. The autonomic nervous system is regulated by the hypothalamus, which forms part of the limbic system in the brain. The limbic system is the part of the brain from which our emotional responses are generated. This means that your emotions can elicit responses from the autonomic nervous system. For example, if you have a fear of heights or acrophobia and find yourself facing the prospect of going to the highest floor in a building, you are likely to experience the fight and flight responses because your anxiety will create the stress situation that activates the body to fight or flee.

This means that the involuntary responses are not limited to external stimuli or factors but can also be triggered by internal factors such as our emotions.

Involuntary responses can be primarily characterized as either fight or flight responses or rest and digest responses. Fight or flight responses, as we have seen, prepare our bodies to cope with stressful situations by increasing the energy levels available to the cells, tissues, and organs in the body. The system that initiates or regulates the fight or flight responses is the sympathetic nervous system.

The sympathetic nervous system stimulates the adrenal glands which, in turn, release catecholamines such as adrenaline and noradrenaline. In response to the release of the adrenaline and noradrenaline, sympathetic fibers in the spinal nerves use the neurotransmitter noradrenaline to activate increased blood flow in the lungs and in the skeletal muscles. This released in an increase in respiration and heart rate.

The other part of the autonomic nervous system is the parasympathetic system, which functions to inhibit the sympathetic responses of fight and flight in the body. The parasympathetic system is responsible for rest responses in the body. It helps the body to conserve energy by slowing down the heart rate, relaxing sphincter muscles, and increasing gland activity. This system promotes digestion and the synthesis of glycogen, and in effect, facilitates normal function and performance in the body.

Parasympathetic fibers are typically found in the cranial nerves and use acetylcholine as the main neurotransmitter to initiate their rest responses. The parasympathetic nerves originate from the nuclei in the brain stream and branch into the cranial nerves, including the facial nerve, glossopharyngeal nerve, the Vagus nerve, and the oculomotor nerve.

The vagus nerve functions in the regulation of the heart rate through the innervation of the cardiac muscles while the oculomotor nerve is involved in the constriction of the pupil. Responses such as salivating, tearing of your eyes, digestion, urination, or sexual arousal are all triggered by the parasympathetic nervous system.

Ultimately, the sympathetic and parasympathetic systems have opposing functions in the body, and they both need to regulate each other's responses in order to keep the body in a balanced state. When you are in a state of danger, your flight or fight responses are activated by the sympathetic system. Once the threat has been resolved, the parasympathetic system takes over and inhibits the fight or flight responses bringing the body back to a rested state.

When there is dysfunction in the functions of the sympathetic and or parasympathetic systems, this will cause physiological and physical disorders. For instance, when the sympathetic nervous system is overstimulated without being inhibited by the parasympathetic system, then disorders such as chronic inflammation and autoimmune disorders can arise.

In summary, the main distinctions between the sympathetic and parasympathetic divisions of the autonomic nervous system are:

Sympathetic Nervous System (SNS)

- Responses: Fight or flight
- Spinal cord distribution: Thoracolumbar
- Preganglionic neuron: Short
- Postganglionic neuron: Long
- Neurotransmitter: Noradrenaline

Parasympathetic Nervous System (PNS)

- Responses: Rest and digest
- Spinal cord distribution: Craniosacral
- Preganglionic neuron: Long
- Postganglionic neuron: Short
- Neurotransmitter: Acetylcholine

Functions of the Nervous System

Sensation

We interact with our surroundings using our senses of touch, sight, sound, smell, or taste. Once we come into contact with an external stimulus using any of our senses, a signal is sent to the nervous system which receives the information from the environment, and in effect, helps us register what is going on around us. Our senses of touch and sound enable us to detect physical stimuli while taste and smell senses detect chemical stimuli. Our sense of sight detects light stimuli.

Consider what would happen if you were crossing the rail tracks and could not hear the oncoming train? Or if you could not tell if your bath water is too cold or too hot? Our senses enable us to interact safely with our environment by enabling us to detect potentially harmful stimuli so that we can respond appropriately. Without proper function of our sensory organs, our brain cannot accurately interpret or recognize what we are exposed to.

Response

Timmy is bouncing a ball in his backyard and humming happily to himself. He pauses for a while to take off his shirt. He is sweating quite profusely, but he is determined to enjoy the beautiful summer day. As he wipes the sweat on his forehead, he spots a butterfly flying from one leaf to the next. He drops his ball and starts running after the butterfly, his little arms outstretched as he tries to scoop it up.

In this simple scenario, we can see how we first sense our environment and then respond to what we are seeing. In this case, Timmy sees a butterfly, and once he spots it, he decides to run after it. Our response to the environment is based on the ability of the nervous system to sense and identify what has been sensed so that we can respond appropriately to it. In Timmy's case, had he seen a snake instead of the butterfly, his response would have been to run away from it, not towards it.

Once we come into contact with external stimuli, a signal is sent to the brain to enable us to recognize what we are seeing, and then this is followed by a reaction that will depend on the stimulus that has been detected. The function of the nervous system occurs in a continuous loop that starts with the sensation of the stimuli, then to perception or identification of the stimuli, and finally, the response to the stimuli.

The cells that facilitate the communication of the signal from the sensory organ to the nervous system are neurons. They relay the signal from the detected stimulus to the brain via the spinal code, where the process of identification or perception occurs. In the final step of the process, the neurons transmit the signal from the brain to various glands and muscles to elicit the appropriate response.

Responses in the body can either be voluntary (which occur on a conscious level), or they can be involuntary (which occur on a subconscious level). Voluntary responses are usually brought about by the contraction of skeletal muscles and are regulated by the somatic nervous system.

When it comes to involuntary body responses, they are characterized by the stimulation of glands, regulation of the heart muscles, and the contraction of non-skeletal muscles which are also referred to as the smooth muscles. Involuntary responses are regulated by the autonomic nervous system. Sweating is an example of an involuntary response; it occurs automatically without conscious effort.

Integration

Once we have interacted with a certain stimulus, we need to understand what it is before we can react to it. This function of the nervous system, where the information obtained from the environment through our senses is processed, is called integration.

The integration process consists of the comparison of the information being received with previous stimuli that we have identified in our memories and past experiences. This comparison enables us to recognize and categorize stimuli that we have interacted with before. For example, when you first encounter poison ivy, you may not be aware that it will have a burning sensation on your skin, but the second time you come across it, you will automatically stay away from it because your nervous system will be able to identify it as a harmful stimulus.

Consider a child who has been burned by the stove; they will always be wary of it from that point on because they have already had an experience that can be used to classify the object as dangerous. This integration process thus determines how we categorize experiences, whether pleasurable or harmful, and ultimately, how we respond to the stimuli we are in contact with.

The Cranial Nerves

The peripheral nervous system is part of the nervous system. It connects to various body organs through the cranial nerves and spinal nerves. The cranial nerves originate from the brain and exit the skull at its base. Cranial nerves contain sensory and motor neurons, though some cranial nerves only have sensory neurons.

There are 12 paired cranial nerves, all with different functions. These nerves are:

I	The Olfactory nerve which controls our sense of smell
II	The Optic nerve which regulates vision
III	The Oculomotor nerve which regulates the movement of the eyeball and eyelids.
IV	The Trochlear nerve which regulates eye movement
V	The Trigeminal nerve which controls chewing and facial sensations.
VI	The Abducens nerve which controls eye movement.
VII	The Facial nerve which controls our facial expressions as well as our sense of taste.

VIII The Vestibulocochlear nerve which regulates balance and hearing.

IX The Glossopharyngeal nerve which controls the secretion of saliva, sense of taste, and swallowing

X <u>The Vagus nerve</u> which regulates smooth muscles and motor responses in the heart lungs and throat.

XI The Accessory nerve which regulates neck and shoulder movement.

XII The Hypoglossal nerve which controls speech, tongue movement as well as the swallowing mechanism.

The Optic nerve, olfactory nerve, and the vestibulocochlear nerves are all sensory nerves. They regulate our vision, smell, and hearing senses. For instance, the lack of hearing would indicate a problem with nerve VIII, the vestibulocochlear nerve, which regulates our hearing and equilibrium. The optic nerve controls both our peripheral and central vision, while the olfactory nerve regulates our sense of smell. The olfactory nerve can be tested by closing your eyes and one nostril and then using the other to inhale different scents and checking to see if you identified them correctly.

Movement of various body structures is under the control of the motor nerves. Motor nerves include; oculomotor, trochlear, abducens, hypoglossal, and accessory nerves. Speech, tongue movement, and swallowing functions are controlled by the hypoglossal nerve. The accessory nerve, on the other hand, regulates shoulder and neck movement, while eye movement is controlled by the oculomotor, trochlear, and abducens nerves.

There are cranial nerves that have both sensory and motor functions, and these nerves are referred to as mixed nerves. The Vagus nerve, the trigeminal nerve, the glossopharyngeal nerve as well as the facial nerves are all mixed nerves with both sensory and motor functions. The largest cranial nerve is the trigeminal nerve, which is composed of ophthalmic, mandibular, and maxillary nerves. The trigeminal nerve regulates facial sensation, corneal responses as well as chewing.

The facial nerve functions in both controlling facial expressions and our sense of taste. The symmetry of the face or lack thereof can be used to test the facial nerve. The swallowing mechanism, sense of taste, and secretion of saliva all fall under the control of the glossopharyngeal nerve. Motor control of the digestive system and smooth muscle sensory in the heart, lungs, and throat are all regulated by cranial nerve X, which is the Vagus nerve.

Chapter 2

The Vagus Nerve

The Structure of the Vagus Nerve

The Vagus nerve is the body's primary parasympathetic nerve. It supplies parasympathetic fibers to all the body organs including the major organs such as the heart and lungs. It is the key pathway for the transmission of information between the brain and other body organs and tissues. The vagus nerve, as a result, enables the brain to monitor functions of various body organs and systems in the body.

The 10th cranial nerve (Vagus Nerve) is the longest and most complex of the 12 cranial nerves. It originates from the brain and runs through the face, neck, chest, and abdomen. The Vagus nerve is a mixed nerve meaning that it has both sensory and motor functions, and as such, plays a crucial role in facilitating effective organ to the brain communication and brain to organ communication. Due to its extensive length and pathway from the brain to other body organs, it is also referred to as the wandering nerve.

From the medulla of the brain stream, the vagus nerve exits the cranium through the jugular foramen, which is located in the base of the skull. Within the skull, the auricular branch of the Vagus nerve arises to provide a sensory response to the auditory canal as well as the external ear. From the head, the vagus nerve then extends to the neck through the carotid sheath.

The vagus nerve, while in the neck, will travel inferiorly with the jugular vein and the carotid until the base of the neck, at which point, the right and left vagus nerve branch into two different pathways. The right vagus nerve enters the thorax by passing anteriorly to the subclavian artery and posteriorly to the sternoclavicular joint. In contrast, the left vagus nerve will enter the thorax, passing posteriorly to the sternoclavicular joint and between the carotid and left subclavian arteries.

While in the neck, the Vagus nerve branches into:

- **The superior laryngeal nerve** consists of internal and external branches. The external branch of the laryngeal nerve provides sensory innervation for the larynx through the cricothyroid muscle. The laryngopharynx is innervated by the internal laryngeal nerve.

- **The pharyngeal branch** which provides motor innervation to muscles of the soft palate and pharynx.

- **The recurrent laryngeal nerve** extends from the right subclavian artery to the larynx and function in innervating the muscles of the larynx.

Once the vagus nerve gets to the chest area or thorax, it branches into the posterior vagal trunk and the anterior vagal trunk. The anterior vagal trunk arises from the left vagus nerve, while the posterior vagal trunk arises from the right vagus nerve. The smooth muscles of the esophagus are innervated by the esophageal plexus, which is formed by these vagal trunks.

The cardiac branches, which also arise in the thorax, function in the innervation of the heart muscles regulating the heart rate. Most of the muscles of the larynx are innervated by the left recurrent laryngeal nerve. The vagal trunks from the thorax extend to the abdomen through an opening in the diaphragm, referred to as the esophageal hiatus.

While in the abdomen, the vagal trunks divide into multiple branches that supply the small and large bowels, the stomach, and the esophagus.

The Functions of the Vagus Nerve

Our brain does not just react to external stimuli to keep our environment safe and conducive for us, it also requires constant communication with other body organs. Communication between the brain and other body organs serves to ensure the optimal functioning of the various body systems is maintained. Body organs require regulation such that processes can be activated or inhibited depending on the situation or physical state of our bodies.

If, for instance, you are jogging, your body will require more oxygen to facilitate the increased demand that is occasioned by physical activity. For this to happen, the heart and breathing rates need to increase, so that more air is pumped by the lungs and blood circulation is enhanced to increase the supply of this oxygen to the tissues and muscles. This ability of the body to regulate functions and maintain homeostasis is crucial for normal function and our overall health and wellbeing.

The Vagus nerve plays an important afferent role by bringing information from the internal organs such as the heart, lungs, and gut to the brain. However, it also functions in an efferent role where it mitigates the effects of the sympathetic nervous system.

The Vagus nerve, in its parasympathetic role, acts in contrast to the sympathetic system. It has an inhibitory effect on the sympathetic system, such that when it is activated, it inhibits the fight and flight responses of the sympathetic system. For example, while the sympathetic system will cause the constriction of blood vessels, the parasympathetic system, when activated, will have the opposite effect and cause dilation of blood vessels.

The Vagus nerve, which is the 10th cranial nerve, has both sensory and motor functions in the body. The sensory functions of the vagus nerve can be visceral, which are the sensations in body organs or somatic which are the sensations in the muscles and skin.

The sensory functions of the vagus nerve include:

- Supplying visceral sensation to the heart, lungs, digestive system, trachea, esophagus, and the larynx.
- Providing somatic sensation to parts of the throat and the ear canal.
- The sensation of taste at the base of the tongue

The motor functions of the vagus nerve include:

- The vagus nerve stimulates heart muscles, which, in turn, facilitates regulation of the heart rate.
- The vagus nerve facilitates the movement of food through the digestive tract by stimulating contractions in the esophagus, stomach, and in the intestines.
- The vagus nerve stimulates muscles in the larynx, pharynx, and in the soft palate.

To accomplish body homeostasis, the vagus nerve functions in its parasympathetic role and inhibits the flight or fight responses initiated by the sympathetic nervous system in response to a threat or stressful situation. Let's say that you encounter a wild hog while out hiking in the woods. Once your brain registers the existence of this threat, your fight or flight responses will be instantly activated to enable you to either fight this threat or run away from it. All these responses are initiated to enable you to neutralize the threat and avoid possible harm.

Let's look at a different situation, where you have to do a public presentation and the idea of speaking in public is making you apprehensive and panicky. In this case, your body will activate the sympathetic responses of fight or flight to help you cope with this stress. Regardless of whether you are facing a physical threat or a perceived emotional threat, your sympathetic responses will not distinguish between physical and mental stresses and will react in the same way by initiating the fight or flight response.

The mode of action of the sympathetic responses of fight or flight is to basically increase the energy available to the body to enable it to fight or flee from a particular threat. This increase in energy is achieved by increasing your heart rate, which means blood is pumped at a faster rate and also increasing your respiration such that your breathing becomes quicker.

Now, imagine if you were constantly in a state of agitation as in the case of someone suffering from chronic stress, this would mean that your fight and flight response would be constantly activated. This means that you would have an accelerated heartbeat, increased rate of respiration, and inhibited digestive function for prolonged periods of time. This would definitely take a toll on your physical health by, among other things, elevating your blood pressure, damaging your cardiovascular muscles, and inhibiting proper digestive function.

When the sympathetic system is not effectively counteracted by the parasympathetic system, the constant fight or flight responses will start to cause physical disorders by the overstimulation of certain functions. This is why the vagus nerve in its parasympathetic role in the nervous system is so important for optimum health. It ensures that the sympathetic responses are not active for prolonged periods of time unchecked.

The vagus nerve effectively puts the body back in a relaxed or rested state by slowing down the heartbeat, decreasing the rate of respiration, and stimulating digestive function. These interventions by the vagus nerve ensure that once a threat has been resolved, your body is reverted to a relaxed and rested state. This relaxed state is what creates a conducive environment for the body to engage its self-healing mechanism, prevents chronic inflammation, and mitigates against chronic stress and anxiety.

Without the effective functioning of the vagus nerve, the sympathetic nervous becomes overstimulated, and this, in turn, causes organ malfunction. To ensure that our vagal tone is high, there are measures we can take to routinely activate its parasympathetic effects and ensure that we reap the benefits of its self-healing power. We can activate the vagus nerve using various techniques such as meditation, exercise, breathing techniques, cold therapy, and many other techniques.

The Role of the Vagus Nerve in Good Health

Cardiovascular Health

The vagus nerve functions in the control of our heart rate, in effect, acting as a natural pacemaker. By stimulating heart muscles, it can effectively slow down our heart rate when it is too fast as happens in stressful conditions. When the heart rate is increased, it can lead to elevation of the blood pressure, which causes strain on the heart tissue and blood vessels.

By lowering the heart rate, the vagus nerve effectively reduces blood pressure, and by extension, reduces the pressure on the cardiac muscles. A properly functioning vagus nerve is, therefore, crucial for cardiovascular health and in avoiding conditions such as hypertension.

Prevention of Inflammation

When out tissues get infected, the body responds to the attack by activating the immune system, which dispatches white blood cells to the scene of infection to neutralize the threat.

These responses result in inflammation, which is characteristic in cases of physical injury or illness.

However, when an inflammatory response triggered by the immune system is prolonged, it causes the body to start attacking its own cells resulting in chronic inflammation. Chronic inflammation leads to autoimmune conditions such as rheumatoid arthritis.

The vagus nerve is able to effectively control inflammation by inhibiting the overstimulation of the immune system that is caused by the sympathetic nervous system. Medical research has shown that stimulation of the vagus nerve helps in resolving conditions related to prolonged inflammation of tissues in the body.

Breathing

Our ability to breathe is controlled by our lungs, which are regulated by the Vagus nerve through the neurotransmitter acetylcholine. Proper breathing is not only an effective way to deal with pain but is also effective in coping with stress by creating a calming effect on the body.

Relaxation techniques such as meditation

and yoga incorporate breathing techniques because proper breathing has a relaxing effect on the body.

Improved memory

Stimulation of the vagus nerve has been found to have an effect on improving memory. This is accomplished through the neurotransmitter norepinephrine being released into the amygdala, which forms part of the limbic system. This means that the activation of the vagus nerve can be beneficial in counteracting the effects of some cognitive disorders.

Weight management

Communication in the gut-brain axis is facilitated by the vagus nerve. When the vagus nerve function is impaired, it loses the sensitivity that enables it to detect fullness in the stomach. When the vagus nerve cannot send a message to the brain that the stomach is full, it means you will not be able to know when you are full or not, and this is likely to cause overeating.

Stimulating the vagus nerve increases its sensitivity to the fullness signal from the stomach, and this increased sensitivity will cause you to feel fuller faster and, as such, will result in reduced food intake.

Stress management

When the body's sympathetic responses have been activated, we go into flight and fight mode. One of the characteristics of being in fight or flight mode is the release of the stress hormone cortisol. Cortisol is a stress hormone released by the adrenal glands. The sympathetic system triggers the release of cortisol in response to various stress factors.

However, when cortisol levels remain elevated for prolonged periods of time, it has a myriad of harmful effects, including weight gain, high blood pressure, insomnia, and chronic fatigue. The vagus nerve, with its parasympathetic effects of inhibiting sympathetic responses, can effectively inhibit the release of cortisol by putting your body back into a rested and relaxed state. It is for this reason that people with a stronger vagus nerve response recover faster from illness or stress.

Gut feelings

Have you ever been walking on a dark street and felt the hairs on the back of your neck stand up? Or just met a person and had an instinctive response that you could not really explain? Well, that is called a gut feeling, and though many of us regard them as fancies or whims, gut feelings are actually very real. The gut is capable of conveying your feelings to the brain through the vagus nerve in the form of electrical impulses. This communication facilitated by the vagus nerve through the gut-brain axis is vital to our mental health as it impacts how we behave.

Chapter 3

The Polyvagal theory

In 1994, Dr. Stephen Porges of the University of Illinois advanced the polyvagal theory. This theory stipulates that the nerve has a distinct hierarchical model of three subdivisions. These are:

- The dorsal vagal division
- The sympathetic system
- The ventral vagus system

The dorsal vagal system

The dorsal vagus nerve is a large nerve that extends from the brain through the spine to the lungs, heart, and stomach. It is present in all animals and plays a role in sleep and relaxation by:

- Moderating the heartbeat
- Moderating breathing
- Aids in food digestion

In essence, the dorsal vagal maintains a balance between arousal and relaxation states in the body. However, when the sympathetic functions of the nervous system are overstimulated, the dorsal vagus nerve can shut down, and this will effectively send our bodies into a 'freeze state.'

We have seen an animal freeze in its tracks in the presence of danger; think of coming upon on a deer while driving at night. It may become so frightened that it simply freezes and becomes immobilized on the road staring into the headlights. Possums have also been known to get into a 'freeze' state in the presence of danger only to become reanimated when they feel safe again. But have you ever wondered how this comes about? After all, animals are not intelligent enough to 'play dead,' or are they?

As we have established, the autonomic nervous system has sympathetic and parasympathetic functions. When we are in situations of danger or stress, our sympathetic system kicks in to facilitate fight or flight responses that we use to safeguard ourselves from harm. We seek to resolve our stress or dangerous situations by either fighting or fleeing.

If you encounter a vicious dog, you can react in one of either two ways: pick up a stick and fight the dog or run away from the dog.

However, if our mechanisms of fight or flight fail in resolving the stress, the sympathetic system can become overstimulated to such an extent that our bodies are unable to handle it. Once this happens, the effect will be that to counter the overstimulation of the sympathetic system, the parasympathetic system responds so strongly that it sends the body into a "frozen" state.

This "freeze" state is what results in immobilization, dissociation, emotional detachment, or even the inability to think clearly. This "freeze" state can be short term, as in the case of the possum, which reanimates once the threat has passed or can last for a long time or even indefinitely.

The sympathetic system

As we have explored in the previous chapter, our sympathetic system is part of the autonomous nervous system that enables the body to react in response to stimuli. This system controls our fight and flight responses and acts on the following body organs:

- The heart - it increases the heart rate
- The lungs - increases respiration through

bronchiole dilation

- The gut- causes constriction of gastrointestinal muscles and organs
- Blood vessels- it causes dilation of blood vessels to increase blood flow
- The eye – causes pupil dilation
- Sweat glands – stimulates sweat secretion
- Kidney – inhibits the secretion of renin
- Penis- inhibits erection
- Digestive tract – inhibits food movement along the tract(peristalsis)

These effects serve to prime the body for action by increasing access to energy reserves, improving heart and respiratory functions, and enabling us to either fight or flee from threats. These stress reactions offset the rest and relaxation effects of the parasympathetic system. In effect, the sympathetic and parasympathetic system works to create a balance in the function of internal body organs and achieve a homeostatic state in the body.

The Ventral Vagus System

The polyvagal theory stipulates that the third division of the vagus nerve function is the social engagement parasympathetic system that is attributed to the ventral vagus nerve. This nerve is present in mammals that raise their young, and it typically goes to the facial muscles.

The ventral vagus system is myelinated to increase and control the speed of reaction and responses. This nerve is also referred to as the smart vagus due to its influence on our adaptive and prosocial behavior. Individuals with a greater vagal tone have been found to have a greater aptitude when it comes to social engagement and adapting to different social situations.

The ventral vagus system has inhibitory effects on sympathetic stimulation on the heart, meaning that when the ventral vagus is active, it creates a calming effect that is conducive for social engagement. When you are anxious, or under emotional stress, you are less likely to feel like socializing or emotionally connecting with others because, in your agitated state, you will not be receptive to social interaction. The ventral vagus system, by counteracting and inhibiting the sympathetic effects on our body organs, creates a feeling of calmness, which tends to soothe us into a positive mood and emotional state.

The vagal tone is used in psychological medicine and research to analyze the physiological precursors of various disorders. A diminished vagal tone has been found to result in complications that may impact an individual's ability to respond effectively to stress. Stressful events naturally disrupt our physiological state, which, in turn, impacts our behavior. Emotions, stress, and social behavior can, therefore, be linked to our capacity for social communication and self-soothing behaviors that enable us to effectively exit extreme fight or flight states that result in a 'freeze' state.

The hierarchical structure of these three divisions of the vagus nerve, as postulated by the Polyvagal theory means that they function in a natural sequence or order depending on the situation. When we are in a safe environment and are nor feeling threatened in any way, we use our ventral vagus system meaning that we are calm, express our emotions freely with facial expressions, and use a modulated voice pattern.

On the other hand, when we perceive a threat or hazardous situation, then the sympathetic function of the nervous system kicks in and triggers our flight or fight responses. If we are able to resolve the stress, we will gradually go back to a relaxed state. However, if the stress is not fixed, then the overstimulation of the sympathetic response will cause us to go into the "freeze" or shutting down state that is facilitated by the dorsal vagus nerve. In both the fight and flight mode and the freeze mode, our capacity to engage socially is diminished and inhibited to a great extent.

Chapter 4

Disorders Associated with Vagus Nerve Malfunction

For proper organ function as well as cell and tissue health within the body, the internal environment has to be stable and relatively constant. This stable internal environment is called homeostasis and is the ideal state for organ function. For homeostasis to be achieved in the body, the sympathetic and parasympathetic branches of the autonomic nervous system have to function in equilibrium such that they can cancel out each other's responses. An imbalance between the sympathetic and parasympathetic systems can result in disorders and conditions in the body where organ and tissue functions are disrupted by the imbalance.

The vagus nerve, therefore, plays a major role in the maintenance of body homeostasis by inhibiting fight and flight responses and reverting the body to a rested state. The vagus nerve, which is the tenth cranial nerve, functions in parasympathetic responses both in motor and sensory pathways. Not only is it connected to all the major organs such as the heart, lungs, and gut, but it also plays a role in boosting the overall body immunity. Ultimately, when the vagus nerve is not functioning properly, we become susceptible to both physical and psychological disorders.

Symptoms of Vagus Nerve Dysfunction

The function of the vagus nerve in the parasympathetic system and its effect on key organs in the body such as the heart, lungs, and gut means that this nerve plays a critical role in our overall health and wellbeing. The vagus nerve is the largest cranial nerve and has both sensory and motor functions. It stems from the brain traveling down through the neck and thorax all the way to the abdomen. This means that the vagus nerve is an important afferent and efferent pathway for the communication from the organs to the brain and from the brain to the organs.

The effect of the vagus nerve on the heart rate, breathing, and digestive function means that it is important to have this nerve functioning at optimum levels if we are to maintain proper organ function as well as optimum mental health. Some of the symptoms that can be associated with poor functioning of the vagus nerve include:

Gastroparesis

This condition affects the ability of the stomach to empty itself by affecting the contractions that move food along the digestive tract. This condition can result in bloating, blood sugar fluctuations, vomiting, loss of appetite, or abdominal pain.

Vasovagal syncope

There are some stress factors that can result in the overstimulation of the vagus nerve. Stresses such as exposure to extreme heat or phobias can cause an overreaction from the vagus nerve, which results in a significant drop in heart rate and blood pressure resulting in fainting where a person passes out for a while.

Since the vagus nerve is widely spread out through the body with sensory and motor effects on various tissues in the body, when it ceases to function properly, there is undoubtedly a myriad of symptoms that arise. The symptoms that will manifest will be dependent on part or section of the vagus nerve that is affected. Some of the common symptoms of malfunction of the Vagus nerve include:

Chronic fatigue

Fatigue is the feeling of exhaustion, both physically and mentally and is usually characterized by an overall lack of motivation and energy. While it is ordinary to feel weary after a long day at the office or intense physical activity, chronic fatigue is characterized by a lack of energy and feeling of general malaise that cannot be attributed to one particular cause.

If you are suffering from chronic fatigue, you will find that you tend to feel tired, even first thing in the morning, just after waking up. You experience a sluggish feeling that stays with you throughout the day, and you may even be prone to feeling you do not want to do anything at all. If you find yourself constantly feeling tired, with little energy, and no motivation to face the day even when you have just woken up, you might need to check the health of your vagus nerve. Infection of the vagus can lead to an individual developing chronic fatigue.

Irritable bowel syndrome

The vagus nerve plays a significant role in enabling digestive functions, and when it is not working properly, abdominal disorders become a possible symptom. The inflammation of the cells lining the digestive tract due to prolonged fight or flight response activation can lead to bowel irritation.

When the vagus nerve is doing its job properly, it mitigates inflammation by inhibiting sympathetic responses. However, when the vagus nerve is malfunctioning, the sympathetic responses become prolonged, leading to inflammation.

The vagus nerve innervates the muscles of the gut to facilitate the movement of food along the digestive tract, thereby enabling digestion. This function is, however only possible when the body is in a rested state. This means that if your vagus nerve is unable to switch off the flight and fight responses, the body remains in an agitated state meaning that digestive functions are impaired, which ultimately results in irritable bowel syndrome.

Anxiety

Life is full of ups and downs. From work-related pressure, relationship problems, and family dysfunction, there are multiple experiences and situations that cause anxiety to the ordinary person. In most cases, you should be able to deal with anxiety as it comes and goes. However, if you find that you exist in a constant state of anxiety, this may be an indicator that your vagus nerve is not functioning properly.

It is the role of the vagus nerve to restore the body to a relaxed state and facilitate self-soothing that ensures that we are not constantly agitated. Stresses activate our sympathetic responses, which equip us for flight or fight by priming our bodies for action. For your body to revert to a rested state from this state of agitation, the vagus nerve parasympathetic responses need to override the responses initiated by the sympathetic nervous system.

This means the vagus nerve should be able to slow down your heart rate and breathing rate so that you can feel calm and relaxed. If this parasympathetic mechanism of the vagus nerve does not work properly, you will be prone to chronic anxiety which, in turn, can result in chronic inflammation or even depression.

Chronic Inflammation

Chronic inflammation is typically an indication that our immune system is overstimulated, and as a result of its prolonged action, the body starts fighting its own cells resulting in chronic inflammation. When your vagus nerve is functioning properly, it can switch off the prolonged response of the immune system by preventing the secretion of the tumor necrosis factor and stimulating the release of acetylcholine. These two mechanisms, when instigated by the vagus nerve, are effective in inhibiting inflammation. This, however, is only possible if the vagus nerve is functioning properly.

Chronic inflammation can lead to serious physical and mental disorders., and increasingly, Vagus nerve therapy is being used to mitigate the effects of inflammation in diseases such as Rheumatoid arthritis and epilepsy.

Heartburn

The hypersensitivity to acid reflux is referred to as heartburn. We have all, at some point, experienced that burning feeling in our throats after eating certain kinds of food. This burning sensation is typically our body's response to excessive acid in the digestive tract.

The vagus nerve plays a vital role in the communication between the gut and brain, and if this communication pathway is disrupted, the regulation of the gut can be impaired, which can result in the accumulation of acid and heartburn as a result.

Inflammation

Nature has equipped us with natural defense mechanisms that safeguard us from harmful external threats and internal stresses such as infections. These mechanisms are not limited to just humans or animals but are also evident in plants.

Ever wondered why roses have thorns or why poison ivy has a burning effect when touched? This is nature's way of safeguarding the plants from external threats to ensure their longevity. In plants, defense mechanisms can vary from the thorns on a rose flower to the resin compounds secreted by the poison ivy to keep threats away. Ultimately, the goal is to limit the susceptibility of the plant to an external attack by equipping it with a self-defense mechanism.

In humans, our internal defense mechanisms are facilitated by the nervous system and the immune system. We are susceptible to different kinds of attacks as humans. We can suffer from infections caused by disease-causing microorganisms such as bacteria or viruses. When you have a cold, it is usually a result of a viral infection. Pneumonia, flu, sore throat, and bronchitis are all common ailments that result from pathogenic infections.

The immune system functions by identifying pathogens in the body and eliminating them. This means that our ability to fight off and recover from infections is dependent on the capacity of the immune system to identify and eliminate the disease-causing pathogen. Pathogens are foreign antigens that invade our cells and disrupt normal cell function. Microorganisms such as bacteria, viruses, and fungi are common pathogens that invade the body.

The role of the immune system is to use its constituent cells, such as the white blood cells, to identify and eliminate pathogens from the body, in effect restoring cell function to normal. For the immune system to function properly, it needs to be able to identify its own cells and differentiate them from foreign or invading pathogens.

One of the methods that the immune system uses to identify and fight infection by pathogens and heal itself is inflammation. An inflammatory response is triggered by the immune system to aid in the healing of wounds or infections from pathogens or tissue damage. Inflammatory reactions such as swelling when you hurt yourself or redness of a wound or secretion of pus are a sign that the body is fighting the infection by mobilizing white blood cells to the site of infection. Without inflammation, healing of wounds, infections, and tissue damage would be impossible.

Inflammation can either be acute or chronic, depending on what caused it and how long it lasts. Acute inflammation is short-term inflammation and may be caused by tonsillitis, physical damage such as cuts and scrapes on the skin, bronchitis, or a sore throat. Typically, these conditions will last for a few days or a week, so the inflammation is not prolonged.

Chronic inflammation, on the other hand, occurs when inflammation is protracted and lasts for a long period of time, ranging from weeks to months or years. Some of the cases that are characterized by chronic inflammation include:

- Asthma
- Rheumatoid arthritis
- Periodontitis
- Tuberculosis
- Chronic peptic ulcers

Chronic inflammation can result from an overactive immune system response to an infection, pathogens, or foreign antigen remaining in the body for extended periods or from pathogens that the body cannot break down. Chronic inflammation is usually slow in onset and lasts for a long time, and may ultimately result in tissue death or scarring of connective tissue.

When our sympathetic responses are over-activated, or our immune system is overactive causing it to affect the cells in our own bodies, this can result in inflammation. The immune system has critical functions in the body in terms of fighting off infections and enabling us to recover from illnesses. However, when an immune response is protracted, it starts to cause self-harm to the body by targeting healthy cells in much the same way it would invading pathogens.

If the immune system is not inhibited effectively by the parasympathetic nervous system, chronic inflammation can cause disorders in tissues and organs and ultimately impact the physical and psychological health of the individual.

The Role of the Vagus Nerve in Inflammation

While a certain level of inflammation is essential after physical injury or infection to enable the healing process, prolonged inflammation has a detrimental effect on the body and may cause complications and disorders arising from tissue damage. Autoimmune diseases such as rheumatoid arthritis occur when the body, through the immune system, starts attacking its own cells.

The vagus nerve, with its parasympathetic roles in the nervous system, aids in inhibiting the effects of overactive immune responses such as chronic inflammation by detecting the presence of cytokines and the tumor necrosis factor that is produced by the immune system. Once these compounds are detected, the vagus nerve signals the brain, and this signal initiates the production of anti-inflammatory neurotransmitters such as acetylcholine.

The vagus nerve also acts through the splenic nerve to curb the release of the tumor necrosis factor by macrophages, and in this way, functions to reduce and inhibit inflammation in the body.

Physical disorders

Rheumatoid Arthritis

Rheumatoid arthritis is an autoimmune disorder that is caused by chronic inflammation that leads to tissue damage in the joints. It is characterized by swollen joints, joint pain, the development of rheumatoid nodules, limited range of motion in the affected joint, and in extreme cases, may result in joint deformity.

Vagus nerve inhibition of cytokine production serves to reduce inflammation, and this has been found to be effective in providing symptomatic relief for rheumatoid arthritis patients. When inflammation is reduced, then the swelling in the joints and the pain can be significantly reduced, meaning that the patient can experience relief from the symptoms of rheumatoid arthritis.

Vagus nerve stimulation in Rheumatoid arthritis patients has been found to have a significant impact on the secretion of the tumor necrosis factor. When the tumor necrosis factor is actively being secreted, it causes inflammation, and thus by inhibiting its production, the vagus nerve is able to reduce the levels of inflammation in the body, which results in a reduction in the severity of rheumatoid arthritis.

Stimulating the vagus nerve is, therefore, an effective management therapy of conditions that arise from chronic inflammation such as rheumatoid arthritis.

Inflammatory Bowel Disease

Inflammation of the digestive tract is typical in illnesses such as Crohn's disease and ulcerative colitis. Crohn's disease can be triggered by inflammation of the lining along the digestive tract and may spread into deep tissues of the bowel. Crohn's disease leads to the development of symptoms such as abdominal pain, diarrhea, weight loss fatigue, and even malnutrition in extreme cases.

The development of Crohn's disease has been linked to factors such as malfunctioning of the immune system and genetics. Though most who suffer from Crohn's disease may not have a family history of the disease, genes have been found to play a role in increasing susceptibility to the disease. A protracted immune response to infections has also been found to be a possible cause for the development of Crohn's disease.

When you have a bacterial infection in the digestive tract, the immune response produced may be too protracted. In this case, the immune cells start attacking even the cells that form the inner lining of the digestive tract. When this happens, the inflammation and damage of the cells lining the digestive tract are inevitable.

Vagus nerve stimulation can relieve inflammation by inhibiting the effects of an overactive immune response. A non-drug therapy targeting the anti-inflammatory pathway of the Vagus nerve has been found to ease inflammatory systems in colitis and inflammation of the digestive tract. The high tumor necrosis factor characteristic in inflammatory bowel diseases can also be inhibited by the parasympathetic function of the vagus nerve.

The vagus nerve can prevent peripheral inflammation by initiating the release of glucocorticoids through the activation of the hypothalamic-pituitary-adrenal. Additionally, the release of Acetylcholine effectively inhibits the production of the tumor necrosis factor, which is a factor for inflammation.

Diabetes

The primary source of energy in the body for cellular functions is blood glucose. When we consume food, glucose is extracted from the food and then broken down in the presence of the hormone insulin to generate energy for various cell functions. The hormone insulin is a necessary component in the breakdown of glucose.

In situations where we have developed low insulin levels or insulin insensitivity, cells are, as a result, unable to access energy from glucose in the blood. This results in hyperglycemia or the presence of excess glucose in the blood, which is brought about by the lack of efficient breakdown of glucose. This condition where there are excess glucose levels in the blood is referred to as diabetes and can occur in two types:

- **Type 1 Diabetes**

In type I diabetes, the immune system attacks cells in the pancreas, which, in turn, interferes and inhibits the production of the hormone insulin. Since insulin is required for the breakdown of blood sugar, once its production is repressed, it then results in an elevation of blood glucose levels because glucose is not being broken down effectively.

- **Type 2 Diabetes**

Type 2 diabetes is mainly caused by the body's inability to use insulin efficiently due to insulin insensitivity or when the body does not produce sufficient amounts of insulin to breakdown blood glucose levels.

Stimulation of the vagus nerve can aid in regulating insulin production by inhibiting overactive immune responses that result in the destruction of the pancreatic cells that function in insulin production. While the immune system is crucial in preventing infections in the body, the overstimulation of the immune system results in the destruction of the body's own cells.

Initiating the parasympathetic responses of the vagus nerve by stimulating it can impede the production of the tumor necrosis factor, which causes inflammation. Additionally, by the production of acetylcholine neurotransmitter, the vagus nerve helps in regulating inflammation.

Vagal stimulation also plays a part in averting cardiac arrhythmias that can result from severe hypoglycemia

Hypertension

The force that your blood exerts on blood vessels is referred to as blood pressure. Hypertension refers to a state in which the blood pressure is elevated higher than what is ideal for good health. High blood pressure can cause a myriad of complications such as stroke, heart diseases, or even kidney failure. It is, therefore, important to ensure that we effectively manage our blood pressure to avoid health complications that may be fatal.

Hypertension has been linked to a lack of adequate physical activity, diet, and poor stress management. When a person is obese or overweight, the heart has to work harder to pump blood, which means that the pressure of the blood being pumped increases, and this creates stress and damage on arterial walls. Poor diet choices that cause thickening or obstruction of blood vessels also increase blood pressure and have adverse impacts on cardiovascular health.

Chronic stress is a major predisposing factor for hypertension. The vagus nerve has a significant impact on stress management, meaning it is equally effective in regulating blood pressure and reducing the chances of hypertension. When our fight or flight responses are activated by the sympathetic nervous system to enable us to deal with emotional or physical stresses, our vital organs are strained by the increased demand for energy in the body. In this stressed state, our heart rate increases, our rate of respiration equally goes up, and our digestive tract functions are inhibited.

If we remain in this state of agitation for lengthy periods, this additional stress on our major organs inevitably leads to health complications such as high blood pressure. When the vagus nerve, which is parasympathetic in nature, is activated, it mitigates the effects of the sympathetic responses by restoring the body to a state of rest and relaxation by slowing down the heart rate, dilating the bronchioles, and stimulating digestive functions. The vagus nerve is, therefore, an important therapy for hypertension through regulation of the heart rate and playing a significant role in stress management.

Gastroparesis

The normal function of the digestive tract requires that the food moves along the digestive tract so that digestion or food breakdown can take place. When food is moving along the digestive tract, nutrients can be extracted from the food and absorbed by the body, and waste products can be efficiently eliminated from the body. These processes are crucial for a healthy abdomen.

Gastroparesis occurs when this process is inhibited, and food does not move along the digestive tract as required. This condition is caused by the dysfunction of the vagus nerve. The muscles in our stomach rely on the vagus nerve to innervate them and facilitate the movement of food through peristalsis. If these muscles do not function properly, then food movement along the digestive tract is inhibited.

Gastroparesis is characterized by symptoms such as bloating, nausea and vomiting, loss of appetite, and weight loss. Gastroparesis makes control of blood sugar difficult and predisposes patients to the formation of obstructions in the stomach that prevent food from passing into the small intestine. Additionally, bacteria can easily grow when food ferments in the stomach.

Stimulation of the vagus nerve innervates the stomach muscles enabling movement of food along the digestive tract. Further, by keeping the body in a relaxed state, the vagus nerve creates a conducive environment for digestive processes, unlike sympathetic responses of fight or flight, which inhibit optimum digestive functions from taking place.

Epilepsy

Epilepsy is a neurological disorder that is characterized by seizures that are triggered by abnormal brain activity. The abnormal brain activity interrupts the normal function of various organs, which results in epileptic patients exhibiting the following symptoms:

- Uncontrollable jerking movements in the limbs
- Staring
- Confusion
- Loss of consciousness

Focal epileptic seizures are caused by abnormal activity in one part of the brain. These types of seizures may result in complete loss of consciousness where the patient becomes unresponsive to their environment, or they may not cause a lack of consciousness but cause involuntary jerking of limbs, dizziness, or alter smells and appearance of objects.

Generalized seizures result from abnormal brain activity in all parts of the brain. They can be in the form of:

- Petit mal seizures typically affect children and are characterized by subtle body movements and may cause loss of consciousness.

- Tonic seizures which affect muscles in the back, arms, and legs

- Atonic seizures that are characterized by loss of muscle control, causing the patient to collapse.

- Clonic seizures affect the facial tissues, neck as well as the arms. This type of seizures typically presents with jerking muscle movements.

- Grand mal seizures can cause an abrupt loss of consciousness, jerking of the body, and tongue biting.

The abnormal brain activity that brings about epileptic seizures may be due to other conditions such as stroke or head trauma. Infectious diseases that target the brain, such as meningitis and prenatal injury, can also result in seizures. Children with epilepsy may outgrow the condition as they grow older, while in some epileptic patients, lifelong treatment is necessary to control seizures.

Vagus nerve stimulation is a therapy used in the treatment of epilepsy that involves the use of a pulse generator to stimulate the nerve into calming and reducing abnormal brain activity, which causes seizures. The role of vagus nerve therapy in epilepsy is in reducing the intensity, frequency, and duration of seizures.

The soothing effect of the vagus nerve helps to tone down abnormal brain activity, ensuring that even when the seizures occur, they are mild and more manageable. While the vagus nerve stimulation therapy cannot cure epilepsy, it plays a significant role in managing seizures when used long term in conjunction with epileptic drugs.

Mental disorders

Chronic Stress

Conflicts, work-related pressure, bills, dysfunction in family or relationships, illness, and so many more factors have made the levels of stress to rise significantly in recent years. Life is challenging in more ways than one, and as a result, stress has become a common part of our existence and daily life.

The human body has developed mechanisms through the sympathetic nervous system branch of the autonomic nervous system to equip us to deal with stress. What most people do not know is that our body responds to both physical and emotional or perceived stress in the same way. This means that a hiker facing a physical threat from a mountain lion and someone having a panic attack because they are afraid of giving a public speech will elicit the same physiological reactions in the body. In both cases, the sympathetic responses of fight or flight will be initiated.

The main role of the sympathetic nervous system is to avail more energy to us when we feel threatened so that we can effectively fight or flee from the threat. To accomplish this, the sympathetic system increases heart rate, respiration rate, and slows down digestive functions.

When you are afraid as, in the case of the hiker facing a mountain lion, or anxious as, in the case of a student about to take an exam, you will notice that your heart tends to beat faster and your breathing is quicker. These sympathetic responses prime you for action and put you in an agitated state with adrenaline coursing through your body.

While this fight or flee responses are vital for our survival, keeping the body for prolonged periods in an agitated state is detrimental because it can lead to cardiovascular disorders, interference with proper digestive function, and cause chronic inflammation. It is, therefore, important for us to manage our emotional stress just as much as we manage physical threats because, ultimately, the effect on the body is the same.

The role of the vagus nerve in stress management is due to its ability to counteract the sympathetic responses and effectively restore the body to a calm and relaxed state. We are often advised to take deep breaths when we are getting angry or about to lose our temper, but have you ever wondered how this simple maneuver helps you stay calm? Deep breathing has been shown to activate the vagus nerve, which through its sensory responses, can innervate heart muscles slowing down our heart rate and gradually restoring the body to a soothed calm state and reducing agitation and anxiety.

Being chronically stressed may be an indicator that your vagus nerve is impaired and that you may benefit from stimulation of the vagus nerve to restore its parasympathetic responses that will enable your body to switch off the fight or flight responses.

Not only is the vagus nerve helpful by physiologically helping us to manage stress, the ventral vagus system boosts our capacity for social engagement enabling us to connect well with other people, which is also a very important factor in stress management. Lonely people are usually more susceptible to stress because they do not have a social network that provides emotional support that we all need to deal with stress.

Alzheimer's

Alzheimer's is a cognitive disorder characterized by loss of memory, impairment of the ability to think clearly, and the progressive loss of behavioral and social engagement skills.

This disorder results from the gradual degeneration and death of brain cells, which, in turn, causes the impairment of brain functions and cognitive abilities.

Alzheimer's ultimately leads to dementia which is a condition referencing the decline in mental function that results in an individual being unable to live and function normally. Alzheimer's presents as a progressive ailment starting with forgetfulness and memory loss and progressing to an inability to perform even simple and straightforward tasks.

Our ability to perform simple physical tasks such as eating or bathing and cognitive functions such as memory, recognition of people and places, or operating machinery and tools is normally wired into our brains. This is why patients developing Alzheimer's will forget even their children's names or where they live and will be unable to do tasks that they were able to do before such as driving. Deterioration of the brain cells inevitably causes us to lose our mental aptitude and erases most of what we know.

Alzheimer's is a distressing condition not only for a patient who, in essence, loses all notion of who they are but also for the family members who watch the gradual deterioration happen and the transformation of a person from an independent functional human being to a helpless person dependent on others. While there is no treatment that can cure Alzheimer's, there are therapies that are used to slow down the degeneration of brain cells.

Neurodegenerative disorders are enhanced by the prolonged activation of the microglia. This chronic activation can cause a predisposition to degenerative diseases such as Alzheimer's and dementia. The vagus nerve stimulation can inhibit the chronic stimulation and aid in slowing down of the neurodegeneration.

Observations on the effect of vagus nerve stimulation on the microglia illustrate a morphological change that deters neurodegeneration in the brain cells. Microglia in patients with chronic inflammation shows fewer and shorter branches when compared to the microglia in a person with a healthy central nervous system where the parasympathetic responses of the vagal nervous system are able to mitigate overstimulation of the microglia.

Depression

Depression is a severe mental disorder that can affect how you feel act and think. Until recently, depression was considered to be just a person experiencing a bad mood or passing anxiety. In actual sense, depression is much more than just feeling low or being in a bad mood. It is a mental state that is characterized by emotional detachment, feelings of sadness or loss, and a lack of interest in activities. Depression is a serious mental illness that has been linked to suicide and destructive social behavior.

Is it possible to determine the cause of depression? While it is not possible to single out a single factor as the main course of depression, social factors, biological, and psychological sources of distress have been found to be predisposing factors that lead to depressive tendencies. This distress that is initiated by a combination of these factors alters and impairs brain function resulting in psychological and even physical disorders.

Depression weakens your immune system leaving you susceptible to infections that your body could easily ward off if you were not depressed. It has also been associated with poor weight management. Have you ever noticed that you tend to either eat too much when you are feeling low or to not eat at all? Depression has an undeniable effect on our weight by causing us to become obese through overeating or underweight by not eating enough. While binge eating after you have had a stressful day will probably not have long term effects on your health, people with chronic depression develop long-term bad eating habits, which ultimately impact their health.

Insomnia, fatigue, and cognitive impairment are also common effects of depression. Indecision and lack of thought clarity are common in people with depression and can be aggravated by other effects of depression such as fatigue and insomnia, which also affect our alertness and ability to focus. Beyond the physical and mental disorders, depression impacts our capacity to engage with others. Depressed people will more often than not withdraw from friends and relatives, become emotionally detached, and lose interest in physical contact, including sexual activity.

Decreased neuronal plasticity and chronic inflammation of the brain may result from chronic depression. Stimulation of the vagus nerve has been shown to inhibit inflammation and help in combating social distress by alleviating anxiety and fear. The vagal branch of the vagus nerve improves our ability to engage socially with others, and in effect, helps in combating the emotional detachment that is associated with depression.

The effects of the vagus nerve responses on stress management are also key factors in helping people recover faster from depression, thereby helping prevent the mental effects of prolonged depressive states. Studies have shown that Vagus nerve stimulation is especially effective in people with treatment-resistant depression. In vagus nerve stimulation therapy for patients with depression, an electric device is fitted in the patient's neck or chest area to enable stimulation of the vagus nerve through electrical pulses.

Adrenal fatigue

Let's face it; we all deal with stressful situations on a daily basis. From a demanding boss, a failing relationship, or even a problem child, day-to-day life is littered with messes that need cleaning up and problems that need fixing. However, when each mishap starts to feel like a life and death situation, then your hormonal balance is likely out of whack.

When the vagus nerve is either overworking or not working enough, the hypothalamus stops signaling the pituitary gland appropriately, which results in overproduction of some hormones and not enough of others. The net effect of this hormonal imbalance that is created in the body is that every problem either starts to feel like the end of the world, or you find yourself not acknowledging real issues that need to be addressed.

These extremes that are triggered by hormonal imbalance can lead to disorders such as insomnia, lack of motivation, anxiety, chronic stress, and fatigue. This condition where the adrenal glands are not able to respond appropriately to stimuli is referred to as adrenal fatigue.

Vagus nerve stimulation can help in keeping your hormonal balance in check and reduce the tendency to get worked up or stressed over small issues that can be resolved.

Chapter 5

Vagus Nerve Stimulation

The thought of going to the hospital or seeking some form of treatment usually feels us with dread. They are synonymous with pain and suffering, and while no one likes going to the doctor, we all get infections or ailments from time to time that requires medical care and treatment. However, there are ways that we can tap into the natural self-healing power of the body and reduce the number of times that we need to seek medical intervention.

Diseases are a natural part of life because our bodies are susceptible to the wear and tear that comes with age as well as infections and physical damage inflicted by pathogens and other stimuli. This means that the quest for good health is a never-ending journey because we cannot escape the inevitable effect of nature and our surroundings on our health.

Whether you find your comfort at the bottom of the pill bottle, or in alternative therapies, our goal ultimately remains the same; to improve our quality of life by staying healthy and avoiding diseases. The quest for longevity has led to the development of research in various aspects of medicine, from disease prevention, diagnosis, treatment, and cure, the winding road to better health has led to important findings that we can use to better our health.

While human advances in medicine cannot be downplayed, it is important to remember that medicine has side effects on the body. When taken for prolonged periods of time, conventional medicine can have adverse effects on our bodies in the form of side effects. While conventional medicine is beneficial for the treatment of various ailments and conditions, we should do the necessary to reduce the incidences where we need to take it and avoid over-reliance on pills and potions.

In an ideal situation, being able to stimulate the vagus nerve effectively will enable the body to become more adept at keeping illnesses at bay, meaning that you will need less medical intervention to stay healthy. The body's self-healing mechanism functions best when the internal environment is in a rested state.

This means that when the fight and flight responses are activated, the body's self-healing mechanism cannot work. Therefore, when you unleash the parasympathetic power of the vagus nerve through stimulation, you effectively shut down the fight or flight responses and activate the body's self-healing mechanisms.

The 10th cranial nerve, which is the Vagus nerve, is the longest nerve in the body extending from the brain through the neck and thorax all the way to the gut. This nerve, with its sensory and motor response functions, has significant roles in the regulation of organs such as the heart, lungs, and gut. The parasympathetic roles of the vagus nerve, which inhibit the effects of the sympathetic nervous system, meaning that the vagus nerve is an important factor for proper organ function and optimum physical and mental health.

The roles of the vagus nerve in maintaining homeostasis and balance in the internal environment of the body have led to the discovery that the vagus nerve can be used not only in boosting our overall immunity but also in facilitating the body's self-healing mechanism.

Now that we can appreciate how important the vagus nerve is when it comes to good health, the next question would be, how do you measure the activity of the vagus nerve? That is where the vagal tone comes in.

Vagal Tone

Vagal tone is the term used to refer to the activity of the vagus nerve. As we have established in the previous chapters, the activity of the vagus nerve has significant effects on:

- heart rate regulation
- vasodilation and constriction of vessels,
- glandular activity in the heart,
- glandular activity lungs
- gastrointestinal sensitivity and motility and
- regulation of inflammation.

When it comes to health, the vagal tone is measured in terms of the consistent nature of the parasympathetic action that the vagus nerve exerts. While the vagal input is constant, the degree of the stimulation it exerts is influenced by various factors including the parasympathetic responses of the autonomic nervous system. This means that the vagal tone will vary depending on the internal environment in the body. For instance, when the body is in a state of fight or flight, then the vagal tone or activity will be diminished.

Vagal tone can be used as an indicator of various organ functions in the body, including cardiac function, and may also be used in assessing emotional regulation or any other factors that can be influenced by parasympathetic responses such as digestive functions.

The measurement of vagal tone is done using either invasive or noninvasive procedures. Measurement of the vagal tone using invasive procedures is characterized by the use of manual or electrical methods to stimulate the vagus nerve. When it comes to non-invasive techniques, the vagal tone is typically determined by the assessment of the heart rate and heart rate variability. Heart rate variability (HRV) is the difference in the time lapse that occurs between heartbeats.

When the vagal tone is high, then the heart rate is typically slower, and on the other hand, an increased heart rate is an indication that vagus nerve activity is diminished. The vagal tone in the body is a useful tool in the determination of emotional, psychological, and even possible physical disorders that may manifest as a result of poor vagal activity or function.

Vagus Nerve Stimulation

The vagus nerve has both afferent and efferent functions in connecting the brains to organs such as the heart, lungs, and gut. This means that it facilitates communication from the brain to the organs (afferent) and communication to the brain from the organs (efferent).

The vagus nerve functions in controlling motor responses in the voice box, diaphragm, heart, and stomach. In addition, it has sensory functions in the ears and tongue. The widespread nature of the influence on the vagus nerve on different organs, therefore, makes it a useful treatment therapy in patients with diseases caused by chronic inflammation, including Alzheimer's, Epilepsy, and Rheumatoid arthritis.

When Vagus nerve stimulation therapy is to be used on a patient, a device that is similar to a pacemaker is implanted in the chest of the patient. A wire from this device is then run from the device to the vagus nerve in the neck by making incisions on the left side of the neck, which allows for the wire to be placed beneath the skin. This device then functions by sending electrical impulses to the vagus nerve which, in turn, transmits these signals to the brain.

These pulses that are transmitted to the brain are used in the treatment of patients with conditions such as drug-resistant depression. The impulses help in battling depression by affecting the circuits in the limbic system of the brain, which is the area that is responsible for our moods and emotions.

In epilepsy, vagus nerve stimulation therapy works in a similar manner. The signals transmitted from the implanted device travel to the vagus nerve, where they are then sent on to the brain. These mild electrical pulses sent to the brain help in controlling the abnormal brain activity that causes epileptic seizures. While vagus nerve stimulation therapy does not cure epilepsy, it plays a big role in reducing the frequency, duration, and severity of epileptic seizures. This therapy has become an important tool in the management of epilepsy.

Perhaps one of the most incapacitating illness, that is caused by chronic inflammation in the joints is rheumatoid arthritis. Not only does it result in severe joint pain, but rheumatoid arthritis also restricts movement as well, and may lead to joint deformities in the long run. This disease is challenging for patients because it severely affects the quality of life by limiting the independence of the sufferer. It has no cure meaning that the patient needs to learn to limit and slow down the degeneration in the joints.

Vagus nerve stimulation therapy has proven to be useful in the management of the inflammation that causes joint degradation, and as such, helping in slowing down the course of rheumatoid arthritis and minimizing symptoms such as joint pain and swelling. When the vagus nerve is activated, it releases acetylcholine and inhibits the production of the tumor necrosis factor from the pancreas.

Both of these mechanisms initiated by the vagus nerve are effective in the reduction of inflammation, and therefore, offer relief in terms of the level of inflammation in terms of swelling, pain, and deformation of the joints. In rheumatoid arthritis, vagus nerve stimulation therapy can be invasive, as in the case of surgically implanting a device to function as a pacemaker or non-invasive where the vagus nerve is stimulated externally.

Vagus nerve stimulation therapy has been used in the treatment of patients with gastroparesis. Gastroparesis is the condition where food movement through the gut is inhibited, resulting in food staying in the stomach too long and blockages being formed. This disease can lead to bacterial infections, abdominal pain, bloating, loss of appetite, and weight loss. Vagus nerve therapy functions by innervating the muscles in the digestive tract that facilitate the movement of food in the digestive system through peristalsis.

These are all classic examples of situations where vagus nerve therapy is used in conjunction with conventional medical intervention to realize quicker treatment or aid in alleviating symptoms that do not necessarily respond to medical pills. However, vagus nerve activation is not only useful for people who are already sick. This nerve can help you in maintaining and improving your physical health and mental state, and as such, we can all benefit from the self-healing powers of this powerful nerve that makes up part of the body's self-healing mechanism.

Activating the Vagus Nerve

The good news is that you do not need to have a device surgically implanted in your body to access the healing powers of your vagus nerve. Your vagal tone is the indicator of the activity of your vagus nerve, meaning that if your vagal tone is high, then the level of activity of your vagus nerve is high, and if the vagal tone is low, then the vagus nerve activity is equally low.

While you might wonder why this vagus nerve is so significant, it is important to realize that in our bodies, like in everything else, too much of anything is detrimental. If you are constantly anxious or revved up in fight or flight mode with a flood of adrenaline coursing through your veins, sooner or later, this will take a toll on your heart, mental state, and overall health.

Conditions such as chronic inflammation, depression, or chronic anxiety arise from an inability to switch off the sympathetic responses and restore calmness and balance in the body. Your vagus nerve is one of your most important tools in achieving a relaxed or rested state that allows our organs, tissues, and body to operate without stress, and hence, achieve optimum functional levels physically, mentally, and emotionally.

Being on the lookout for symptoms associated with poor vagus nerve functions such as chronic stress and anxiety, irritable bowel syndrome, inflammation, insomnia, chronic fatigue, or hormonal imbalance, can give you an indication of whether or not your vagus nerve is functioning properly.

These symptoms, even when they do not directly arise from poor vagus nerve function, can all be alleviated or prevented to a large extent by stimulating the vagus nerve. The vagus nerve equips us to respond to emotional, psychological, and physical symptoms that arise from a lack of balance or homeostasis in the body.

The two arms of your autonomic nervous system, the sympathetic system, and the parasympathetic system are meant to balance out in terms of function to facilitate homeostasis in the body and ensure that the nervous system is working properly. While the sympathetic system is crucial in enabling us to cope with stresses both external and internal through fight or flight responses, the parasympathetic system is crucial in restoring our body back to a relaxed state after the resolution of stresses.

Phases of alertness that are typical in flight or fight responses that are triggered by the sympathetic nervous system are ideally meant to alternate routinely with periods of rest and relaxation that are typically initiated by the parasympathetic nervous system. This balancing act works by ensuring that we do not remain in either a sympathetic/agitated state or a parasympathetic state/relaxed state for too long.

This ideal situation of equilibrium between the parasympathetic and sympathetic systems is, however difficult to achieve because we live in a world where we are constantly faced with emotional, physical, and mental stresses. This means that our sympathetic nervous system is usually constantly activated to help us deal with the constant stresses we encounter on a regular basis.

When the sympathetic system is consistently overstimulated, it means that the parasympathetic system, including the Vagus nerve, becomes inhibited, and thus we need to find ways and tools that we can use to activate or stimulate the Vagus nerve to effectively switch off the sympathetic system.

As we have already established, the vagus nerve is an important part of the parasympathetic system that helps in restoring body function to normal and mitigating the effects of overstimulation of the sympathetic responses which can lead to conditions such as chronic inflammation, depression, poor stress management, and a host of other complications.

Accessing the Healing Power of the Vagus Nerve

Even when your vagus nerve is inhibited by sympathetic responses, they are methods you can use to stimulate and restore parasympathetic responses in your body. Some of these methods include:

1. Diet.

The Vagus nerve is surrounded by a protective sheath of myelin that protects the vagus nerve from injury and ensures that nerve impulses are transmitted properly. Good myelin health is, therefore, important for the proper function of your Vagus nerve.

The health of the myelin sheath, however, starts to deteriorate as we age, meaning that the vagus nerve becomes more susceptible to injury and malfunction the older we get. This protective layer, myelin, is a lipid-based compound, and we can help mitigate the effects of aging on the myelin by observing a healthy diet which should be characterized by:

- **Healthy fats:** Myelin sheath is made up of a fatty layer. This means that eating healthy fats is a good way to keep the myelin around the nerves intact and in good condition. Healthy fats are fats that have good cholesterol such as olive oil, omega 3 fatty acids from fatty fish, and oils from seeds and nuts such as chia seeds.

- **Vitamin C**: This essential vitamin plays a major role in the formation of myelin and enhances the formation of neurons that improve brain function. A diet rich in Vitamin C will, therefore, go a long way in improving your nervous function by ensuring that the vagus nerve is well protected by the myelin sheath.

- Fruits such as strawberries, kiwis, blackcurrants, oranges, guavas, papayas, and lemons are great sources of vitamin C that you can incorporate into your diet. Vegetables such as broccoli, brussels sprouts, bell peppers, and kale are also rich in vitamin c

- **Reduce alcohol consumption**: It is no secret that excessive alcohol consumption impacts brain function. This is partly because alcohol contributes to the degradation of the myelin sheath that protects cranial nerves, including the vagus nerve.

2. Deep breathing

One of the most effective ways to stimulate your vagus nerve is by taking deep breaths and slowing down your respiration rate. Typically, we take between 9 -13 breaths per minute. To stimulate your vagus nerve, you can slow this down to 6 breaths per minute by:

- Inhaling slowly to a count of 6
- Exhaling slowly to a count of 6
- Repeat this rhythm until you feel a sense of calmness.

Deep and slow breathing techniques are effective in slowing down your heart rate. They also act to stimulate your vagus nerve to release Acetylcholine, which is a powerful parasympathetic neurotransmitter that aids in calming the body and restoring it to a rested and relaxed state.

When you feel anxious or stressed out, try this simple breathing technique, and you will be amazed at how effective it is in soothing you into a calm and relaxed state. When the body is in a rested state, psychological and physical health is boosted.

3. Expose yourself to cold/Cold therapy

Cholinergic neurons present in the vagus nerve are activated by exposure to cold. This makes exposing yourself to cold temperatures an easy and effective way to stimulate vagal tone or activity. The cold temperature effectively inhibits the sympathetic responses of fight or flight.

To use cold therapy to activate your vagus nerve, there are various techniques you can use. For example, you can simply turn the water to cold for the last two minutes of your regular shower. Alternatively, splashing ice-cold water on your face will also have a positive effect on your vagus nerve. Taking a walk outside when the temperature is low can also help you activate the vagus nerve.

If you feel that your body is up for the challenge, you can also try taking ice baths. This will involve putting three bags of ice into a half-filled tub and getting in once the ice is melted. To do this safely, ensure that you do not stay in the ice bath for an extended period of time. Taking a hot beverage after the ice bath will be effective in warming you up again.

Cold temperatures have been found to have an effect on reducing stress, anxiety, and stimulating the gastric nerves through vagal stimulation. When you feel yourself getting anxious, losing concentration, or simply getting worn out mentally, splash some cold water on your face or just take a break and walk outside in the cold for a while; it may not solve your problem, but it will definitely calm you down and clear your mind.

4. Chanting

The muscles in your larynx and vocal cords are linked to the vagus nerve. Chanting is a good way to activate the vagus nerve. Using chanting as a mechanism to stimulate your vagus nerve also has a calming effect on the body by helping slow down your heart rate.

To activate your vagus nerve using chanting, the following steps can be used:

- Sit in a comfortable position in a quiet and well-aerated room.
- Close your eyes.
- Have your head, neck, and spine in alignment, but your body should be relaxed not tense.
- Stretch your spine, and as you do so, tilt your chin towards your chest so that your

neck is elongated.

- The elongating of the neck will serve to stretch the vagus nerve.
- Relax your throat so that the vibrations of your chant are distributed around the neck.
- Inhale deeply focusing on feeling the air enter your body.
- Then as you exhale, make the 'Oom' sound without.
- As you chant, do not use force or tense your diaphragm.
- Repeat the inhale followed by the exhale with the 'Oom' sound ensuring that your throat stays relaxed.

Humming and singing are also easy ways to activate your vagus nerve. Ever noticed how good you feel singing in the shower? Well, the secret to the feel-good effect is the stimulation of the vagus nerve. Singing is versatile, and you can do it while stuck in traffic by singing along to your favorite music. Singing is an instant mood lifter and an effective way to activate your vagus nerve and put your body in a relaxed state.

5.Intermittent fasting

Intermittent fasting refers to a nutrition plan where you eat for a certain period of time, followed by a period of abstaining from food, which is the fasting phase. Intermittent fasting means fasting in intervals. For example, you can fast for 18 hours in a day and restrict your feeding period to 6 hours.

When you fast, the vagus nerve detects the inevitable drop that occurs in glucose levels when we go without eating. Once it has detected the drop in blood glucose, the vagus nerve signals the brain to reduce metabolism, which has the effect of slowing down the heart rate and switching of the body's sympathetic responses of fight or flight. In this way, fasting is effective in stimulating vagal activity.

Intermittent fasting has become one of the more popular weight loss methods because it is effective in insulin regulation, and therefore, promotes fat burning in the body. This method, apart from the obvious benefits in terms of weight management, is an effective way to activate the vagus nerve.

If you are trying this method for the first time, an easy tip to incorporate to avoid suffering from hunger pangs is to make your sleeping hours part of your fasting window. For example, you can opt to have your fasting window from 7 pm in the evening to noon the next day, so that most of the fasting period will be used up while you sleep; this means that you will not need to experience hunger throughout the day.

Another great hack for intermittent fasting is ensuring that during the eating window, you consume a lot of proteins as opposed to carbohydrates. This will aid you during the fasting period because proteins are effective as an appetite suppressant. Reducing your carbohydrate intake will also be effective in reducing the blood sugar fluctuations that typically occur between the fasting period and the eating window. Water and non-caloric drinks such as green tea is also a great way to stay hydrated and curb hunger pangs during the fasting window.

To benefit from the effects of fasting in stimulating your vagus nerve, you can opt for moderate fasting plans of 16 hours or 18 hours a couple of times in a week. The ultimate effect is that fasting by stimulating your vagus nerve will also have positive effects on your mental clarity and overall ability to manage anxiety and stress.

6. Physical Exercise

There is no getting away from the fact that physical exercise has multiple beneficial effects on our physical health. It not only improves cardiovascular health; it also helps in fat burning and weight management. Exercise has also been proven to be effective in combating stress and anxiety. When we engage in physical exercise, the body release chemicals called endorphins that have an uplifting effect on the mood and are responsible for the feel-good after effect of exercising.

If that's not enough to get you up and moving, physical exercise is an effective way to stimulate your vagus nerve and enhance your vagal tone. Exercise stimulates your vagus nerve resulting in enhanced mental clarity and stimulation of the brain's growth hormone.

Exercise is a good way to manage stress and boost your immune system. Physical activity stimulates brain function, making you more alert and enhances digestive processes by boosting metabolism and stimulates the movement of food along the digestive tract.

When it comes to stimulating the vagus nerve using physical exercise, there is no limit to the type of exercises you can use. Lifting weights, jogging, taking brisk walks, aerobics, and even yoga will all help in boosting vagal activity and promoting the body's self-healing mechanisms.

7. Massage

Massages can be so relaxing and effective in relieving tension and stress in the body. It is, therefore, no surprise that they can be used as a means of activating the vagus nerve. One of the most effective massages when it comes to vagal activation is reflexology massages.

A reflexology massage involves the application of different amounts of pressure to different parts of the body, specifically, the feet, hands, and ears. A reflexology massage will increase the activity of the vagus nerve, inhibit sympathetic fight or flight responses and even slow down the heart rate. This means that this type of massages soothes the body into a relaxed state that promotes vagal function and mental clarity.

Massaging the neck area is also effective in stimulating the vagus nerve by applying pressure on the carotid sinus. Pressure massages are also effective in vagal stimulation. When you are feeling tense or having a bad day, visiting a good massage therapist will help you to relax and reduce your anxiety and stress levels.

8. Sleep hygiene

Getting enough sleep is important for good physical and mental health. When we haven't slept well during the night, our ability to function well the next day is impaired because we are not rested, and the lack of rest results in a kind of mental fogginess that hinders clarity of thought. Sleeping also allows the body to activate its self-healing mechanisms and rejuvenate itself by renewing worn-out cells and tissues.

When your sleep quality is bad, then your immunity, mental, and emotional health are likely to suffer. The relationship between sleep and vagal tone is cyclic. This means that getting sufficient sleep will boost your vagal tone. On the other hand, when your vagus nerve is not functioning properly, you are likely to experience poor quality of sleep and may even end up suffering from insomnia.

So, how can you improve your quality of sleep? Well, before you reach for the sleeping pills, there are several things you can do to improve your sleep hygiene and as a result, get better sleep quality. These tips are:

- Going to bed at the same time every day.
- Sleeping in complete darkness and

avoiding mental stimulation while in the bedroom, i.e. switch off your gadgets- phones, TVs, laptops, etc.

- Avoid taking naps during the day, if you do take a nap, try to keep it below an hour.

- Do not eat just before going to bed; give your stomach time to settle between mealtime and bedtime.

- Get into a habit of waking up at the same time every day.

- Ensure you get a minimum of 7 hours of sleep daily.

9. Probiotics

The communication between the gut and the brain is facilitated by the vagus nerve through the gut-brain axis. This axis basically links emotional and cognitive brain centers to the gut functions. Our gut plays host to a variety of microbes that are important in enabling the breakdown of compounds during the digestion process. These microbes communicate to the brain using the vagus nerve, and hence the presence of "good bacteria" in our gut is one way of enhancing brain activity.

While the thought of ingesting bacteria may sound revolting, it is important to note that not all microorganisms cause diseases. In fact, most are quite harmless and are actually useful in digestive processes in the gut. Microbes are a natural part of the ecosystem in our gut and actually play a role in improving digestion, preventing infection by hindering the development of disease-causing microorganisms, and boosting the immune system.

Probiotics or friendly gut bacteria play a significant role in:

- Reducing chronic inflammation
- Lowering Cholesterol
- Reducing symptoms of depression and anxiety
- Reducing infections by boosting immunity
- Inhibiting the growth of disease-causing microorganism

The good news is that probiotic-rich foods are easily available and should be pretty easy to incorporate into your diet. They include:

- Yogurt – this healthy drink is made by the

fermentation of milk by gut-friendly bacteria. There are natural and sugar-free varieties available for those watching their sugar intake.
- Sauerkraut – fermented cabbage has been a part of our diet for a long time because even in the olden days, its impact on gut health was well recognized. In addition to its probiotic content, sauerkraut is rich in vitamins such as Vitamins C and K and is rich in iron and manganese.
- Pickles- the fermentation of cucumbers to make pickles makes them a good source of probiotics and vitamins such as vitamin K.
- Cheese – cheese is a favorite addition to many dishes, and cheeses such as cottage cheese, mozzarella, and cheddar are all great sources of probiotics.

10. Yoga and Tai Chi

Both yoga and tai chi have a significant vagal stimulation effect on your body.

Tai chi is a type of exercise that focusses on mind, body, and spirit. It was originally practiced in China though it has now expanded worldwide due to its effectiveness in stress management and weight loss. There are different types of tai chi each with its own methods, but all share common basic principles including:

- Control of movements and breathing
- Generating internal energy
- Mindfulness and serenity

Studies have indicated that tai chi is effective in relieving chronic pain, improving overall body immunity, and promoting physical fitness. If you are seeking a means to activate your vagus nerve that comes with a host of other health benefits, then tai chi might be the way to go. Yoga, similarly to tai-chi, has beneficial effects when it comes to vagus nerve activation and in the reduction of stress and anxiety.

Practicing yoga encourages the mind and body to self soothe and get into a relaxed state, which is the ideal environment for the body's self-healing mechanism to work efficiently. Yoga typically incorporates physical exercise, meditation, and chanting to achieve mental and physical relaxation. There are different types of yoga that can be used to effectively activate the vagus nerve.

11. Good relationships

We have a natural instinct for socialization that is part of the core of the human experience. We actively seek out relationships and connections with others to get a sense of belonging and oneness that is fostered by good relationships. Poor or dysfunctional relationships are one of the leading causes of stress in the world today. Loneliness has, for a long time, been known to create a predisposition to depressive tendencies; this is because human contact is essential for our psychological wellbeing.

Social engagement not only helps us relax, but it also effectively switches off our fight or flight responses by creating a safe and soothing environment for us to exist in. Maintaining good relationships will boost your vagal tone by stimulating your parasympathetic responses and by reducing stress, which tends to activate our fight or flight responses and inhibit vagal activity.

Chapter 6

Meditation

Our body has a natural ability to heal and renew itself. Our cells are capable of continuous self-repair and regeneration. Imagine if all the zits, wounds, and scrapes you have had since infancy had not healed and you were covered in bruises and dents; not a very good picture is it? It is important to understand that our internal organs are susceptible to wear and tear, as well. This means that the body's self-healing mechanism is necessary in keeping cells renewed and in a functional state at all times.

The body's self-healing mechanism is driven by the autonomic nervous system, which facilitates the parasympathetic and sympathetic responses. Sympathetic responses are our bodies' way of responding to threats and stresses. Are you running from a burning building? Are you stressed? Anxious? In all these situations, the sympathetic nervous system is activated and in order to facilitate the fight or flight responses that we need to resolve the threats in our environment.

Consider a situation where the sympathetic system did not kick in when you were facing an imminent threat. There you are, watching this huge dog charging you, and all you can do is stand there transfixed with mouth agape. When you visualize that kind of scenario, it becomes apparent why we need these sympathetic responses. Without them, we would be vulnerable to every danger and threat that comes our way.

The downside to this system, however, is that your nervous system cannot differentiate between when you are being chased by an actual tiger or when you are freaking out over not being able to fit into your favorite pants. As far as the nervous system is concerned, these situations are both threats, and the response elicited is the same, which is basically to switch on the fight or flight responses.

When this happens, the body directs all its energies to functions that are required for fight or fleeing, including increasing the heartbeat to supply more oxygen to the muscles. While this is going on, the body's self-healing mechanism is inhibited and cannot take place until the body reverts to a restive state.

Stress kills, and it does so by impacting on your physical health as well as your psychological state. The fact of the matter is every time you are anxious, depressed, worried, or agitated, your body's self-healing mechanisms are switched off as your body primes itself to either flee or fight the threats you are facing. So, if you want to restore the body's ability to heal itself, what should you do? Well, it's pretty simple; find a way to manage stress and anxiety and activate your vagus nerve in the process.

Living your life trying to avoid pain and stress would be an exercise in futility because while you can control your own actions, you cannot control what others do. Learning to handle stress is a sure way to a healthier body and mind. Fortunately, there are various methods that we can use in destressing and attaining inner peace irrespective of what is going on around us. One of the best techniques for achieving inner peace and mindfulness is meditation.

Increasing Parasympathetic Responses Through Meditation

Meditation is a mental exercise that exercises the mind through relaxation, heightened focus, and creating awareness. Meditation is similar to physical exercise, but for our minds rather than our bodies. Meditation enables us to exercise our minds and purify our thoughts. Meditation is based on the following techniques:

- **Concentration:** This is achieved by focusing attention on a particular object that can be external or internal.

- **Observation:** This is where you concentrate on the sensations, feelings, and thoughts present in your body at that moment.

- **Awareness:** This is where you remain consciously aware of your own thoughts and feelings but without getting distracted or engaged physically or mentally.

Regardless of the type or technique of meditation, the primary goals of meditation are:

- Improving mental awareness and clarity
- Reducing stress and anxiety
- Raising our level of self-awareness when it comes to our bodies, emotions, and thoughts
- Relieving pain
- Achieving inner peace and calmness

All these benefits of meditation soothe our bodies and activate the parasympathetic vagus nerve responses, which, in turn, helps us fight inflammation, irregular brain activity, depression, high blood pressure, and digestive disorders.

Meditation Techniques

Mindfulness Meditation

In mindful meditation, the goal is typically to concentrate your mind on the thoughts, sensations, and emotions that you are experiencing in the present or current moment. It normally involves regulation of breathing, muscle and body relaxation, mental visualization, and a heightened awareness of the body and mind.

Mindfulness meditation is effective in stress reduction, cognitive therapy, as well as in the treatment of depression symptoms. The basic technique involved is easy to learn and can easily be done for about 10 minutes daily to obtain the benefits in terms of increasing your vagal tone.

A simple mindful meditation technique for beginners is described below:

- Find a quiet and well-aerated room to practice your meditation in.

- Sit comfortably on a chair, or you can sit on the floor.

- Ensure that your posture is relaxed and that your shoulder and neck muscles are not tense.

- Your head, neck, and spine should be aligned but not tense or stiff.

- Bring your mind to the present by pulling all your focus to the here and now.

- Concentrate on your breathing, feel the breath enter your body as you inhale, and feel the air exit your body as you exhale.

- Take deep breaths all the time, focusing on the sensation of the rising and falling of your diaphragm.

- To make it easier to focus on your breathing, you can place one hand on your upper chest and the other above your navel. This will aid you in engaging your diaphragm when breathing in and out.

- Breath in slowly through your nose, as you inhale, the hand on your navel area should feel your stomach rise gradually as the air enters your body.

- On the exhale, let the breath out through your mouth with your lips slight pursued. As you exhale, the hand on the navel area should feel the stomach relax and fall back into the starting position.

- As thoughts pop up in your mind, do not quash or try to suppress them; simply turn your attention back to your breathing and focus on the inhale and exhale motions of rising and falling.

- Stay in this state for at least 10 minutes, always pulling your focus back to the present and away from thoughts and emotions by simply focusing on your breathing.

- At the end of the 10 minutes, rise slowly from your position, and allow your mind to become gradually aware of your surroundings.

When you become good at this type of meditation through repeated practice, you will be able to practice mindful meditation without necessarily having to find a quiet room or sit on the floor. The main aim of mindful meditation is to increase your awareness of the present moment by focusing your attention on the now and ignoring thoughts and emotions.

The effect of mindful meditation on your vagal tone is powerful because by reducing stress and inhibiting flight and fight responses that are activated when we are anxious or worried, it allows the body to relax and rest which is the ideal condition for the parasympathetic system to function. Mindful meditation has been found to be effective in reducing inflammation and improving stress resilience.

More benefits of mindful meditation include:

- Increased self-awareness
- Improved concentration and cognitive aptitude
- Better emotional regulation and management
- The overall reduction in stress and anxiety.

Breath Awareness Meditation

Breath awareness meditation is similar to mindfulness meditation in that it encourages you to focus on your breathing as a way of soothing and calming your body. The goal in breath awareness meditation is to concentrate on the breathing motions and sensations and ignore any thought that may crop up in your mind.

A simple technique to follow for this type of meditation involves following the steps outlined below:

- This meditation can be done in an upright or sitting position or even laying down on your back

- You can do this with your eyes closed, or you can leave them open, but your gaze should be down and not looking at anything in particular.

- Feel the muscles on your shoulders the back of your head and neck area. Focus your attention on these three areas.

- Breath in slowly through your nostrils and feel the rise of your shoulders as the air is getting into your body.

- Exhale slowly, and this time, focus on the

falling of your shoulders as the breath leaves your body.

- With each inhaling and exhaling action, feel your jaw, shoulders, and neck beginning to loosen up and relax.

- After a few breaths in and out, begin to think I am breathing in on the inhale and I am breathing out on the exhale. Again, the point of this is to ensure that your mind is entirely focused on your breathing.

- Continue to monitor your breathing for about ten minutes.

- As you come towards the end of the ten minutes, you can stop thinking I am breathing out with the inhale and I am breathing out with the exhale. Allow your mind to stray from the concentration on the breathing.

- While you are exiting this focused concentration on the breathing, ask yourself, "What do I want?" on the inhale and listen to the response from your mind on the exhale.

- Then on the next inhale, ask yourself, "What am I thankful for?' and listen for the answer in your mind as you exhale.

- Acknowledge what you are you are feeling at that moment, open your eyes or bring your gaze back up, and rise from your meditation position.

Transcendental Meditation

Transcendental meditation is a type of spiritual meditation that is mostly spiritually based and focuses on bringing an individual's awareness past their physical being or state. It involves the repetition of particular mantras and the use of particular postures to enhance the feeling of inner peace and calmness. Transcendental meditation differs from mindful meditation in that while mindful meditation is geared towards bringing attention to the present, the aim in transcendental meditation is to transcend or go past thought itself.

In transcendental meditation, you use the repetition of a mantra to settle your mind and remove all thoughts. It does not involve concentration or focusing on a particular object. Transcendental meditation is typically learned from certified teachers because it requires a precise technique to achieve a transcendental state.

The ultimate result of consistent transcendental meditation is an increased awareness of our existence as part of a large cosmos and thus helps in shifting thoughts from our own person to our surroundings and those around us. It is effective in stress and anxiety reduction as well as in creating a high level of cognitive and thought clarity.

Body Scan Meditation

Stress manifests itself in our bodies in terms of tense muscles, shallow breathing, irregular heartbeat, and overall physical discomfort. It is hard to be always aware of how we are feeling each and every time and what is triggering us to feel a certain way.

Have you ever woken up in a bad mood, and you were not even sure why or what was causing the mood? Do you have moments during the day when you feel anxious or agitated for no apparent reason? These are all manifestations of different stresses that take a toll on our emotional and mental health. The problem with stress is that you can become so accustomed to living with it, that you are not even aware that you are stressed until it starts taking a toll on your health.

Body scan meditation primarily involves

examining or scanning your body for areas of tension. The aim is to identify areas where your muscles are tensed or where you have tension knots and essentially relax them to release the tension. The general technique in body scan meditation involves scanning your body from one end to the other. For instance, you can start from toe to head. The following steps can help you in practicing body scan meditation:

- Sit in a comfortable position and relax your body.

- Slow your breathing drown and focus on deep breathing, which is breathing from your stomach, not your chest.

- To help you in breathing from the belly, you can create a mental image of a balloon inflating and deflating in your stomach as you breath in and out.

- Focus on each part of your body, and feel for signs of tension, start from your head and work yourself down systematically through the neck chest abdomen and limbs.

- During this systematic scanning process, keep doing your deep breathing as it will heighten your awareness and ability to detect tension in your muscles.

- Notice the general feeling and sensations in different parts of your body, for instance, if you have soreness, tightness, or tense muscles in any part of your body.

- Once you come across the areas on the body that is tense or uncomfortable, focus on this area as you breathe in and out. You can accompany this focus by gently massaging the area of tension and concentrate on feeling the tension leave your body as you exhale.

- Do this process throughout your entire body, paying special attention to the tense and sore areas until you start feeling relaxed in those areas.

Body scan meditation is very important in increasing your body awareness and your ability to recognize when things are going wrong or not working as they should. This type of meditation is a tool that you can use when you are feeling stressed or anxious, and it will help you in releasing tension and becoming more relaxed.

Like in the other types of meditation, our vagus nerve functions best when we are in a relaxed state, so any type of meditation that helps you relax and get into a peaceful state of mind will be instrumental in activating and stimulating your vagus nerve.

Kundalini Meditation

Kundalini meditation is practiced as part of a type of yoga that focuses on releasing the energy that is present at the base of the spine. This energy is referred to as kundalini energy. In Kundalini meditation, the chief goal is to unleash this power at the base of the spine and using its energy to cleanse your body of ailments, mental and emotional disorders, and essentially purify your system.

For this type of meditation:

- Increase your awareness and prepare your mind to receive the kundalini energy

- Dress in loose, comfortable clothing and find a quiet, comfortable place for your meditation.

- Cover your head using a shawl or scarf

- Sit with your legs folded and ensure that your spine head and neck are aligned but relaxed

- Close your eyes

- Practice deep breathing and focus on the inhale and exhale process

- Break down your inhaling with gaps, i.e. breath in, hold continue breathing in, hold and continue. Inhale this way with four pauses and do not exhale during this step.

- Once you have done the above process, you can then exhale using the same technique, exhale-hold, then continue exhaling, again do these four times.

- Do this staggered inhale and exhale process for about four minutes.

- At the end of the four minutes, inhale deeply, bringing your palms together, and holding them together for approximately ten seconds.

- Then exhale deeply and feel your body relax as you exhale.

- As you continue increasing your breathing rate and feeling the breath in your body, you will gradually be able to control your rate and flow of breath, and as you go deeper and deeper into these breathing techniques, you should start to uncover the energy at the base of your spine.

- Chanting a mantra as you practice your breathing will help in focusing your mind on your body and will also have an overall uplifting effect on you. There is no specific mantra that is required; you just need to find one that speaks to your values or goals and use that as your mantra.

The Wim Hof Method

The vagus nerve is connected to many parts of our bodies, and as such, it has been found that we can activate it naturally using these parts of our bodies to stimulate it. An active Vagus nerve means that our bodies can achieve a state of equilibrium between the parasympathetic and sympathetic nervous systems. When either system is not balanced out by the actions of the other, we tend to develop physical and psychological disorders that impact our quality of life.

The Wim hof method was developed by Wim hof, who has been able to accomplish extraordinary physical fetes such as being submerged in ice for extended periods. The Wim hof method of stimulating the vagus nerve is chiefly based on three main principles, i.e.:

- Cold exposure
- Breathing
- Commitment

Cold therapy

Cold therapy, also referred to as cryotherapy, is one of the pillars of the Wim hof method. Have you ever wondered why a cold compress applied to a bruise or swelling helps in reducing pain and speeds up healing? Applying a cold compress reduces blood flow to a particular area, regulates nerve activity, and results in a reduction of inflammation and swelling.

In the same way, cold exposure has multiple health benefits to the body. It has been found to increase weight loss through fat loss, reduce inflammation, and stimulate the secretion and release of feel-good hormones or endorphins in the body. There are several ways you can expose your body to cold therapy. These include:

- Cold showers - these are an easy way to get cold therapy. You can start off by turning the water to cold when taking your normal shower. As you build up your cold resistance, you can then go for fully cold showers. Not only is a cold show invigorating, but it will also get your vagus nerve activated and energize your mind.

- Ice baths – once you get accustomed to cold showers, you can then graduate to ice baths.

The rule of thumb here is to not subject your body to extremes without first building up your stamina. So, start with the cold showers, and once your body has adjusted and is able to cope with that level of cold exposure, you can then gradually move on to ice baths.

Using about 3 bags of ice, put these in a tub that is half full. And wait until most of the ice is melted, and the temperature of the bathwater is approximately 59 F degrees.

You can start with limited exposure from 5 to 10 minutes, then build up your exposure as your body gets accustomed to the ice water baths. If at any point during bath, you notice your body is getting uncomfortable or is in distress, simply get out as you do not want to cause harm to your body.

After the bath, a hot beverage such as some hot cocoa will help you to warm up. You can also go for a short walk to stimulate blood flow. It is important to remember that cold exposure should be done sensibly and that people with pre-existing conditions should not attempt this kind of therapy to avoid causing complications.

Breathing

Breathing exercises are a tried and tested method of bringing your body and control. From taking deep breaths when you are about to lose it and punch someone in the face to women in labor trying to cope with labor pains, breathing exercises are useful in combating stress and anxiety, minimizing and controlling pain, and restoring your body to a rested or relaxed state. It is, therefore, no surprise that controlled breathing is one of the pillars of the Wim hof method.

Breathing correctly can help in increasing your oxygen levels, slowing down the heart rate, and boosting our body's natural immunity. The basic breathing technique in the Wim hof method can be achieved by following the steps outlined below:

- Sit in a meditation posture with your head, neck, and spine aligned and relaxed.
- Close your eyes.
- Inhale deeply as you feel the air enter your body.
- Hold the breath for a moment.

- Exhale deeply feeling the air empty out completely.

- Inhale again deeply, hold, and then deep exhale.

- Repeat this breathing technique 14 more times.

- After this, you move on to power breaths.

- Breathe in deeply through your nose and exhale through your mouth in short bursts as if you are inflating a balloon.

- Repeat this breathing technique 30 times.

- While doing the 30 inhale-exhale repetitions, practice the body scan meditation technique of going over your body and identifying areas of tension and try and focus your energy on those areas that feel tired or tense,

- After the 30 breaths, inhale deeply until you fill your lungs completely, then again, exhale completely until all the air is pushed out. After the exhale, hold your breath long as you can and focus on feeling the energy in your body as you hold

- After your hold for as long as you can

inhale deeply feeling your chest expand in the process and hold again for about 15 seconds.

- During this hold, try to direct your energy to your tension areas, and mentally picture the tension ebbing away and the negative energy being released.

- Exhale after the 15 seconds hold.

- You can start this technique with one or two rounds of this sequence, and then build up to more rounds as you get more practice with time.

Commitment

Consistency in following your breathing techniques and cold exposure therapies will determine your level of success in improving your mental and physical health.

Rather than starting on a path that you will not be able to follow consistently in the long term, it is better to pick a method that you can easily incorporate into your daily routine. Results in any method take consistency and commitment to follow through. Just like dieting for a day and expecting to lose weight would be unrealistic, following a meditation technique for a couple of days and expecting it to reverse your mental and physical health is not realistic.

Settling on a method that will not strain your physically or in terms of time improves your chances of success because you will be able to stick to the technique long term. So, if you want to hack into your body's self-healing mechanism, take time to select and settle on a method or multiple methods that you can practice regularly and consistently.

Chapter 7

Exercises to Enhance Vagus Function

We all know that physical exercise is a great way to stay healthy, not only does it help you maintain healthy body weight, exercise improves organ functions such as cardiovascular activity, metabolism, and brain activity. Lack of enough physical exercise is a factor in the development of lifestyle diseases such as diabetes, obesity, and heart disease.

Even more important is the role of exercise in stress management and in achieving a healthy mental and emotional state. Ever noticed how good you feel after a workout? This occurs partly because physical exercise triggers the release of feel-good hormones in the body resulting in the uplifting effect that you experience after exercising.

Apart from increasing your energy levels throughout the day, physical exercise is one of the best ways to combat sleeping disorders such as insomnia. Staying physically active during the day ensures that the quality of sleep you get is enhanced. We all know that one of the factors for the development of chronic stress is lack of sleep. So, if you are having a hard time nodding off at night, it may be time to increase the level of physical activity in your daily routine.

The vagus nerve has beneficial effects in battling chronic inflammation, autoimmune disorders, improving gut health, and regulating heart rates, which is essential for cardiovascular health. Apart from physical health, a good vagal tone significantly improves psychological health by promoting stress management. Stimulation of the vagus nerve can be achieved using physical exercises, and perhaps one of the best exercises to achieve vagal stimulation is yoga.

Specific yoga poses

Yoga is a combination of physical, mental, and spiritual exercises that utilizes breathing techniques, exercises, and meditation. The main aim of yoga exercises is to achieve harmony in the body, mind, and environment. Yoga is an ancient art with origins in Asia, which has gained worldwide popularity due to its numerous benefits in terms of mental and physical health.

Some of the benefits of practicing yoga include:

- Management of anxiety and stress
- Decreasing depressive tendencies
- Promoting cardiovascular health
- Increasing self-awareness and self-control
- Improving mental clarity
- Improved balance and body flexibility
- Weight loss
- Muscle relaxation

Unlike other forms of exercise, yoga can be practiced by people at any age because it does not require high-intensity exercise or strenuous activity. Yoga poses can be adapted to suit even the elderly and people with physical limitations. The most important thing is to make sure that you get a credible instructor and that you make them aware of any physical limitations or conditions that you may have so that they can customize the poses to suit your body.

While there are different types of yoga techniques with different poses, it is important to observe the basics before getting started, including:

a) Do not practice yoga on a full stomach.

b) Yoga mats are necessary to prevent accidents and injuring yourself, use a non-slip mat.

c) Remove jewelry, contact lenses, and make sure your hair is tied up so that it doesn't get in the way.

d) It is always important to avoid cramping up and to stretch the muscles before you get started.

e) Find a quiet environment that will enable you to focus on your poses, meditation, and breathing exercises.

Kundalini Yoga

Kundalini Yoga encompasses physical movement, meditation, and breathing exercises to achieve self-awareness. It is a popular type of yoga because of its beneficial results on the mind, and physical health can be realized quickly. Kundalini yoga has been found to be effective in increasing physical awareness and also breaking bad habits.

Instructors of this type of yoga recommend doing it early in the morning and for a period of not less than forty days. A typical Kundalini yoga class will be typically structured as follows:

- the class will start with a 10-minute introduction, and this is accompanied by spiritual teachings from the instructor.
- 45-minute workout, which is also referred to as kriya.
- 15-minute relaxation session also referred to as the Savasana
- 20-minute meditation, which may include the chanting of mantras.

Some of the poses practiced in kundalini yoga include:

➢ Lying down on your back and raising your legs to a 90-degree angle. At the same time, raise your arms and bring them together to interlock above your chest area. Begin by lowering and raising your legs to perform leg lifts. Your arms should remain in the same position. Perform the leg lifts for 9 minutes.

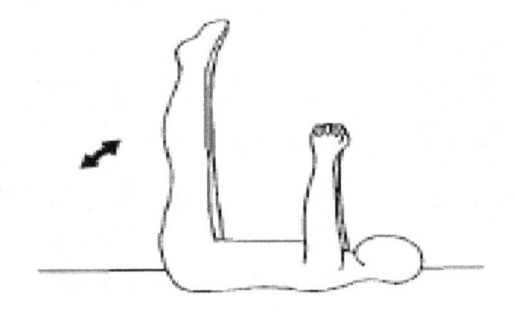

➤ After 9 minutes, stop the movement with your legs raised and hold that position for 90 seconds.

➤ While still on your back, lower your arm and stretch them out above your head. Then resume the leg lifts, raising and lowering both legs for another 90 seconds.

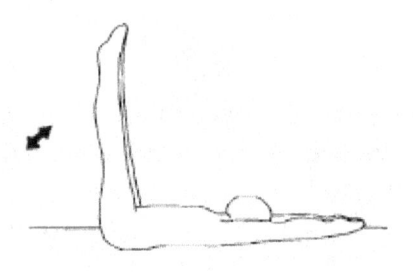

➤ After the leg lift, remain on your back, and with your legs still raised at a 90-degree angle, spread your legs about a foot apart and lower them while spreading them out in this manner. When they touch the ground, bring them together and again raise them to the 90-degree angle, before separating them on the descent.

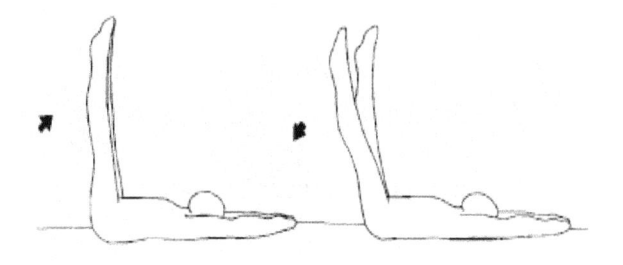

➤ Continue this motion for a minute.

➤ Pull yourself into a shoulder stand.

➤ Bring your knees up and bring your heels to your buttocks. then raise your legs into a handstand. Keep your legs together as you go through these motions.

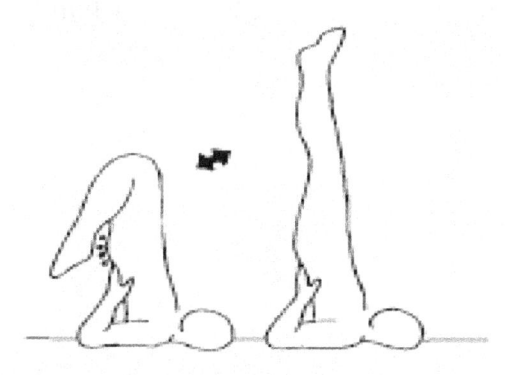

➤ Repeat these motions for 2 minutes.

➢ After the 2 minutes are up, bring your legs down to the floor alternating between the right and the left such that when the right leg is up, the left is down and vice versa.

➢ Begin your chanting as you carry out these alternate leg lifts

➢ Repeat this for about 150 seconds.

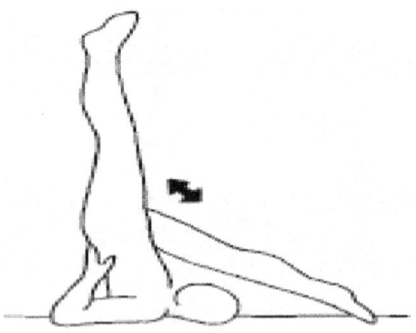

➢ Slowly lower your legs into the plow pose and hold your feet with your hands.

➢ Hold this position for 30 seconds while chanting.

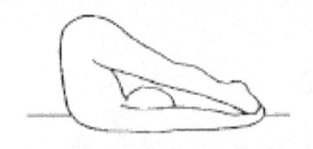

> To finish, lie back down on your back with your legs outstretched. As you get back into the relaxed position, consciously scan your body and focus on the areas of tension as you inhale and exhale.

When it comes to increasing your vagal tone, the role of yoga is to increase the flexibility not just of your body but also of your autonomic nervous system. Yoga can help you in learning how to switch from your sympathetic and parasympathetic systems by mastering stress and recovering from trauma. By following the following yoga practices, you will be able to boost your vagal tone and activate your parasympathetic responses.

Breathing Exercises

Breathing techniques are one of the most effective ways to switch from your sympathetic nervous system and activate your rest and relax responses. The key to deep breathing techniques is to feel the inhale and exhale motions in your upper belly rather than in the chest area. Effective breathing, when it comes to stimulation of the vagus nerve, should also focus on reducing the number of breaths taken per minute and extending the exhale.

Normally, we breathe an average of 11 times per minute. To effectively slow down the heart rate, you need to bring this frequency down to 6 times and focus on longer inhales and exhales. For instance, you can breathe in to a count of 5, hold, then exhale to a count of 8-10. The point here is to breathe deeply, but also to make the exhale longer than the inhale.

You can start off within an even count for the inhale and exhale, and then build up to a longer exhale. For instance, start by breathing in to a count of 5 and exhaling to a count of 5. Repeat this for about a minute, then switch to inhaling for a count of 4 and exhaling to a count of eight. As you keep increasing the length of your exhale, you will get better and better at controlling your breathing.

Another simple but effective way to boost your vagal tone as you go through your exercises is to stimulate the vagus nerve using your facial muscles. Remember that the muscles in your face are also linked to the vagus nerve. Engaging a smile as you go through your motions not only relaxes your jaw and facial muscles but also stimulates your ventral vagus, which is responsible for our social engagement tendencies.

Yoga poses that open up your chest and your heart, so to speak, are also effective in improving your vagal tone. A simple heart-opening pose is bringing your hands to your shoulders while seated. Inhale as you open your elbows wide by pushing them towards your back, then bring your elbows back together in front of your chest as you exhale. Ensure that your breathing is deep during these motions.

The vagus nerve is connected to your gut, and using poses that stretch your stomach area can help in stimulating it. You can stretch your belly using these simple poses.

- Get into a table pose position; this means that you are on all fours with your hands beneath your shoulders and your knees underneath your hips in a kneeling position.
- Inhale slowly and simultaneously lift your head and hips and move into the cow pose.
- Exhale slowly while simultaneously lowering your head and hips and lift your spine into a cat pose

Repeating this motion will stretch your stomach muscles and spine, effectively stimulating your vagus nerve.

Restorative yoga is a great way to calm the nervous system and inhibit sympathetic responses from getting overactivated. Yogic sleep, which is also referred to as yoga Nidra is a great way to relieve anxiety and stress and relax your body. It can be done by lying down in a comfortable position on your yoga mat. Then simply concentrate on your breathing and focus your energy on the tense parts of your body. Remain still in this position for about half an hour. This simple exercise should leave you feeling relaxed and calm.

Useful Tips

Your body has powerful self-healing mechanisms that you can tap into by activating the vagus nerve. While we have looked at the techniques that you can use to access this healing power, the following takeaways will help you in achieving your optimum vagal tone.

Keep your stress levels in check

When it comes to activating your vagus nerve, stress will be your number one enemy. We have already established in previous chapters that for the parasympathetic systems to become activated, your body needs to be in a relaxed and rested state otherwise, your body's self-healing mechanism cannot be activated. Chronic stress keeps you in a constant state of fight or flight and inhibits the vagus nerve from functioning properly.

To avoid being constantly stressed, you can use any of the tools we have discussed, such as meditation, exercise, yoga, or even socially engagement. When you allow stress to dominate your life, the vagus nerve activity is overridden by the fight and flight responses that are activated when we are stressed. Managing stress can be an uphill task, but once you develop this skill, it will be one of the best things you can do for your body in terms of physical and mental wellbeing.

Breathe

We all take breathing for granted, after all, we are all born with the ability to do it, and you have gotten by so far without using any particular technique. It is important to note that breathing is one of the pathways to better health and controlling our nervous system functions. Deep breathing can help you calm down when you are anxious or stressed. It can make the pain more bearable, and more importantly, it can help regulate your heart rate.

If you are ever in a state of panic with your heart beating furiously in your chest, simply taking deep breaths will help you to slow down your heart rate. Paying attention to your breathing is a technique used in meditation because it helps you focus on the present and become aware of what is going on in your body.

Breathing exercises are great because you do not need a special time frame, equipment, or location to perform them. You can simply do them as you go about your normal business and repeat them as many times as you need during the day.

Disease Management

Chronic diseases such as rheumatoid arthritis, Alzheimer's, or epilepsy have no cure. However, stimulating the vagus nerve can help in making them more manageable and bearable for patients. The power of the vagus nerve in inhibiting chronic inflammation and turning down overactive immune responses means that it can greatly slow down degeneration in disorders such as arthritis and Alzheimer's.

In epilepsy, vagal stimulation therapy is now widely used in regulating the frequency, severity, and duration of seizures. This means that if you are suffering from any of these chronic illnesses, you can ask your doctor about including vagal stimulation therapy in your treatment plan to help alleviate some of the symptoms.

Weight Management

When your brain is not able to perceive fullness in the stomach, the natural consequence will be that you will tend to eat more. The communication between the gut and brain is facilitated by the vagus nerve, which means that if your vagus nerve is not functioning properly, your hunger and fullness cues will not be received correctly by the brain.

Activating the power of your vagus nerve can, therefore, help you in weight management by curbing overeating and facilitating proper digestive processing of food in the gut.

Emotional Stress Counts as a Threat

When it comes to responses, your autonomic nervous system only has two options to throw at you, fight or flee or relax and rest. Why is this important to remember? Because we keep on activating our sympathetic system even when we are not aware of it. Think of it this way. Whether you are running from a charging dog or stressed out about a relationship or work, your sympathetic responses will be the same because to the central nervous system, a threat is a threat, whether it is physical or emotional.

Keep emotional stress to a minimum by using any of the stress management techniques we have discussed, such as yoga, deep breathing techniques, or meditation.

Inflammation

Chronic inflammation is usually a sign that our sympathetic responses are over-activated or that our immune system is overactive, causing it to affect cells in our own bodies resulting in inflammation. When the immune system is activated for too long, it can start destroying the body's own cells, and this is what will cause chronic inflammation. If the immune system is not inhibited effectively by the parasympathetic nervous system, chronic inflammation can cause disorders in tissues and organs impacting physical and mental health.

Being on the lookout for signs of chronic inflammation can, therefore, enable you to determine if your vagus nerve is functioning properly. When your vagus nerve is functioning properly, it means that parasympathetic responses can be switched on to inhibit prolonged immune system activation.

Social Engagement

Good relationships are great for your immunity in terms of fighting off diseases and infections and are also vital for your psychological and emotional health.

Establishing great social networks and sound relationships with your family and friends will significantly decrease depressive tendencies and improve your overall ability to cope with stress, which, as we have seen is a big factor in physical and mental disorders.

Research has proven that people with better relationships are happier, healthier, and live longer. The ventral vagus nerve, which is our social engagement or "smart" nerve, improves our ability to connect with others emotionally and enables us to develop socially acceptable behavior and emotional reactions.

Conclusion

Thank you for making it through to the end of the *Vagus Nerve*. Let's hope it was informative and able to provide you with all of the tools you need to tap into the power of the vagus nerve and stimulate your body's self-healing mechanism.

Understanding how your body works and how you can reach your goals in terms of maintaining a healthy body is a great way to tap into the body's potential for self-healing and self-regulation. The sympathetic nervous system and the parasympathetic system balance each other out in order to create a balanced internal environment in the body.

Constant illness and disease can have a huge impact on our quality of life. When we are constantly unwell both physically and psychologically, our productivity, ability to engage with others, and capacity for stress management are all greatly diminished. Accessing the power of the vagus nerve through stimulation gives you back the power to take charge of your health and ensure that your body is functioning at its best.

When we fully understand the power of the Vagus nerve and the significance of its parasympathetic responses in the body, we can then begin to unleash the ability of the body to heal itself and use this as a way of boosting our immunity, enhancing our cognitive abilities, and improving our emotional health.

The vagus nerve plays a big role in our overall health and is one of the major pathways we can use to ensure that we do not suffer from avoidable conditions and disorders. By taking the initiative to learn how the vagus nerve can be activated and its significance to your health and well-being, you have started to good health.

The next step is to start applying the techniques that you have learned in this book and following the guidelines provided consistently to achieve the best vagal tone possible which will, in turn, translate into numerous health benefits for you.

Did you like this book?

☆☆☆☆☆

Tell us with a review on **amazon!**